American Medical Association
Physicians dedicated to the health of America

Building and Implementing Physician Practice Web Sites

Michael A. Rothschild, MD

AMA press

Building and Implementing Physician Practice Web Sites

Internet address: www.ama-assn.org

This book is for information purposes only. It is not intended to constitute legal or financial advice. If legal, financial, or other professional advice is required, the services of a competent professional should be sought.

Additional copies of this book may be ordered by calling 800 621-8335.
Mention product number OP318200.

ISBN 1-57947-155-2

BP38:0160-00:6/01

Contents

Preface

"May [you] live in interesting times."

Ancient Chinese curse,
as quoted by Senator Robert F. Kennedy

This book grew out of the lectures I frequently deliver about Web site creation and the online marketing of medical practices. I have broadened the scope of information to cover a wider range of topics related to the design and development of an Internet presence for individual physicians and medical group practices. I hope this text will be useful for those who are newly considering such a presence, as well as for those who have already made some headway into the development of a practice Web site.

A number of the chapters in this book focus on marketing efforts. As of this writing, the majority of physicians with Web sites use them to raise community awareness about the skills, procedures, and unique benefits offered by their practices. Although there is considerable interest in the medical Internet industry in more ambitious Web-based projects—such as the use of online medical records, connectivity with third-party payers, and telemedicine—these have yet to be explored by more than a small fraction of physicians. Furthermore, the legal, ethical, and technical standards relevant to these projects are far from mature. Therefore, such use of the Internet will not be discussed in depth.

This book assumes that the reader has access to the World Wide Web, but no extensive experience with computers or the Internet is anticipated. As this book is a publication of the American Medical Association (AMA), I expect that the audience will largely consist of those working in the United States health care system. Although the majority of Internet users are in North America, it should be kept in mind that the Internet's global reach frequently results in new contact between disparate cultures. In the field of medicine, this can be a good thing, as it enables American doctors to broaden their perspective on health care as it is implemented around the world. I hope that readers will find this book to be a useful aid to their participation in the online world, doctor-patient communication, and consumer education.

Acknowledgments

I would like to thank the many people who have been a help to me in the writing of this book, and in the creation of the lectures that led up to this project. Marsha Mildred and Katharine Dvorak, my editors from AMA Press, have been extremely helpful in the planning and production of the manuscript. My colleagues and teachers in the field of e-health have been a great resource over the years, including Dr Ron Kuppersmith, Dr John Buenting, Dr Matthew Howard, Ms Cynthia Bissell, Dr Perry Miller, Dr Henry Swett, Dr Ron Konrad, Dr Rodney Lusk, Mr John Rodrigues of the American Academy of Otolaryngology–Head and Neck Surgery, and Dr Michael Johns, editor of the *Archives of Otolaryngology–Head and Neck Surgery*. Mr Rafe Scheinblum of Fastnet and Mr Jon Fallet of Duke University have also been extremely valuable as expert advisors from the industry.

There are several other people in my life whom I must thank. My wife, Jennifer, has always helped me to communicate clearly and succinctly, with her keen perspective, her insightful reading, and her skillful copyediting. My sons, Adrian and Dylan, have been very understanding about the time required for this project, and have always been an inspiration to me. My grandfather, Dave, who was far ahead of his time, gave me my first programmable calculator in 1976, and inspired me to learn how to use it. Finally, my parents have made this and my every other achievement possible: my mother, Naomi, who is growing to love the Internet, and my father, Carl, who surely would have.

New York, NY
March 2001

About the Author

Dr Michael Rothschild completed his undergraduate and medical degrees at Yale University. He trained as a resident in otolaryngology at Mount Sinai Hospital in New York, and subsequently was a fellow in pediatric otolaryngology at the Children's Hospital Medical Center in Cincinnati, Ohio. On the faculty at Mount Sinai since 1994, Dr Rothschild holds joint appointments to the departments of otolaryngology and pediatrics. He is currently an associate professor at the School of Medicine and the director of pediatric otolaryngology at Mount Sinai Hospital.

Dr Rothschild has been involved with computers in medicine for many years, having worked as a programmer in a bioengineering laboratory as early as 1981. Since that time, he has developed software in the field of medical artificial intelligence, as well as CD-ROM–based patient simulation for medical training. Most of his recent work in this field has been related to the medical Internet.

Over the past few years, Dr Rothschild has authored a number of articles and book chapters on the use of computers and the Internet in medicine. He is the online editor for the AMA journal *Archives of Otolaryngology–Head and Neck Surgery*. He has also served as the chairman of the Internet Working Group for the American Academy of Otolaryngology–Head and Neck Surgery from 1997 through 2000, and is currently the chairman of the Academy's technology infrastructure committee. He has been a member of the advisory boards of a number of other organizations such as the International Online Journal of Otorhinolaryngology–Head and Neck Surgery and OTOHNS.net. He has also designed or consulted on the design of Web sites for a number of national medical societies.

Dr Rothschild lectures frequently on ethical and legal issues related to Internet medicine and on the online marketing of medical practices. He has been invited to speak in a wide variety of national and international forums. In addition, he has been providing free online consultation in his specialty through his public service Web site (www.Kids-ENT.com) for the past 2 years. During this time, he has engaged in online exchanges with patients and their families around the world on thousands of occasions.

Chapter 1
Goals of Marketing in the Practice of Medicine

"We grew up founding our dreams on the infinite promise of American advertising. I still believe that one can learn to play the piano by mail and that mud will give you a perfect complexion."

Zelda Fitzgerald, 1932

Marketing is one of the world's oldest professions. Even in the earliest of human societies, the ability to distinguish oneself and to convince others of one's superior qualities was an important skill. As civilization and trade developed, advertising techniques evolved to facilitate commerce. This process was greatly amplified by the evolution of technology and the emergence of a succession of mass media, from print to radio to television and the Internet. Effective marketing—in one form or another—is a vital part of virtually every successful commercial, political, cultural, or social venture.

Expanding Your Medical Practice

Some physicians may look with condescension on the marketing professional, feeling that advertising is somehow lacking in professional dignity and beneath them. However, there is nothing inappropriate about developing or expanding a medical practice by reaching out to prospective patients and referral sources.

The physician is one of the original small businessmen. Doctors were using advertising techniques to build their practices and enhance their income long before fierce competition between medical centers for scarce managed care dollars resulted in the current generation of costly and elaborate radio and television campaigns (Figure 1.1). The physician just starting out in practice needs to make potential referral sources aware of the skills and training he or she brings to the community, and the established academic specialist has a vested interest in maintaining a steady flow of patients to support a center of excellence.

Figure 1.1

A 19th-century physician's advertisement as it might appear had the World Wide Web been available. (Courtesy of the National Library of Medicine. www.ihm.nih.gov.)

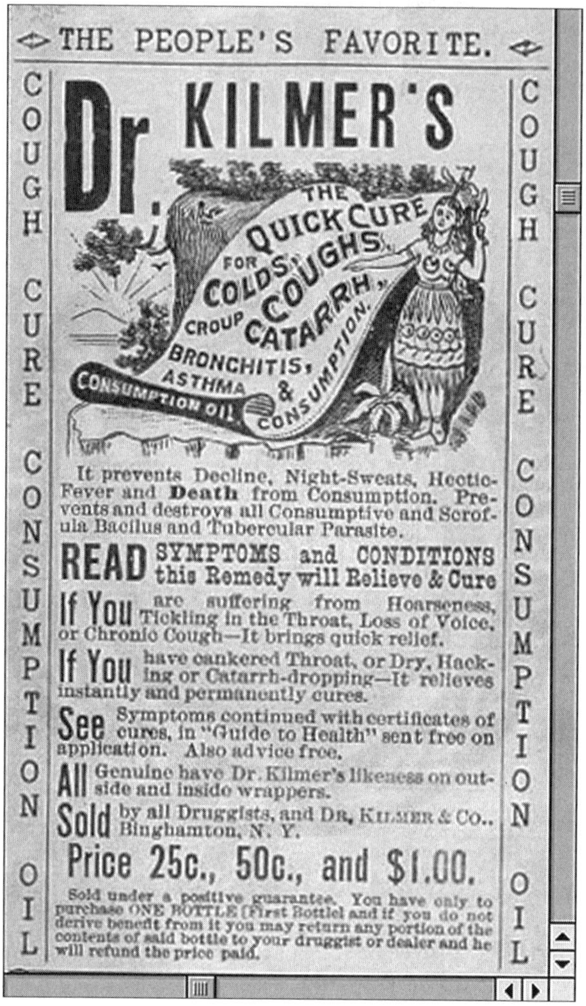

It is true that aggressive advertising campaigns often imply that the seller's motives are purely economic. While this is not a problem for many businesses, it is clearly an undesirable implication in the marketing of medical practices. Even in today's world of big-business medicine, doctors strenuously avoid giving the impression that there is a connection—whether explicit or subtle—between revenue and the level of patient care. This is one of the patient's worst fears: that a physician does not have his or her best interests in mind at all times but is rather "selling" something to them like any other vendor.

There is no shame in being reimbursed fairly for your time, skill, and training, or for accepting the liability and responsibility of patient care. Furthermore, marketing allows for practice building and the appropriate flow of referrals. As long as care is taken to ensure that no hint of unethical behavior or conflict of interest exists, marketing has been and will continue to be an important part of almost any clinical practice. However, before turning to the specifics of online marketing or considering the best way to establish a Web presence, the physician should first analyze exactly what sort of integrated promotional efforts are appropriate. This premarketing analysis is essential to ensure that scarce resources are not wasted. Of course, such an analysis is closely tied to an assessment of the overall goals of the practice, the payer mix, the nature of reimbursement, and the type of care provided.

Assessing Marketing Needs

The first assessment must be a determination of the practice's goals. For a new physician just entering practice, one can assume that the primary goal is to establish a good reputation in the community and to build a patient base. If the physician is joining a busy group, this might not be a problem even in a fully developed market (such as an urban center or affluent suburb). Generally, groups do not add associates unless the current physicians are working at or above capacity, and a steady flow of patients would be provided by internal referral while the new physician's reputation is building. Similarly, a physician starting a practice in an underserved area should not have too difficult a time building a patient base. In this case, marketing would be fairly straightforward, consisting of a notification sent to existing practices or possibly to the community in general.

A more difficult venture is to set up practice in a highly competitive environment, especially without the benefit of joining an established practice. Such a situation calls for relatively aggressive marketing, with emphasis on the unique skills and training the new physician brings to the community. The goal is to differentiate this practice from that of other providers in the same field. More personal contact with referring physicians would be appropriate, and maintaining good communication back to these referral sources is, of course, vital.

Prior to any marketing venture, online or conventional, it is imperative to assess the current needs of the community and the current position of the regional competition. Projected growth of the potential patient base as well as any anticipated expansion in services provided by competing practices should be considered. It is best to define the value that your practice provides to patients, preferably in the form of a fairly simple message that spotlights the unique services you can provide.

Determining the Marketing Target

The nature of the practice determines the marketing target. For some capitated primary care practices, the "selling" is primarily to the insurance companies, and the marginal value of an additional patient may be fairly low. Such practices generally do not spend a lot of time or money in traditional marketing ventures. Other practices, such as those of general surgeons, surgical specialists, or subspecialists in medicine and pediatrics, may be reimbursed in a fee-for-service arrangement according to a negotiated discounted fee schedule in a mature market with extensive managed care penetration. These physicians do have an interest in bringing in additional patients, although the return for each new patient may not be great. Marketing in such a situation is usually directed toward primary care providers who will be the source of new referrals, or toward other specialists when tertiary care referrals are appropriate.

Practices built on a nondiscounted, fee-for-service model may have the largest potential financial return from a marketing venture. Furthermore, a practice in which referrals are primarily patient-driven puts less emphasis on the traditional determinants of referral patterns between doctors and more on the efficacy of the marketing campaign. The classic example of such a situation is cosmetic surgery, in which a single new surgical patient may cover the costs of an entire marketing campaign. For this reason, many of the first online medical marketing ventures were directed toward these practices (Figure 1.2). Cosmetic surgery is well suited to Internet marketing as in many cases outcomes can be easily assessed by potential patients (Figure 1.3). Before-and-after pictures—as traditionally provided in photo albums in the waiting room—are easily posted online provided the appropriate consent is obtained.

Figure 1.2

A Web site for a cosmetic surgery practice.

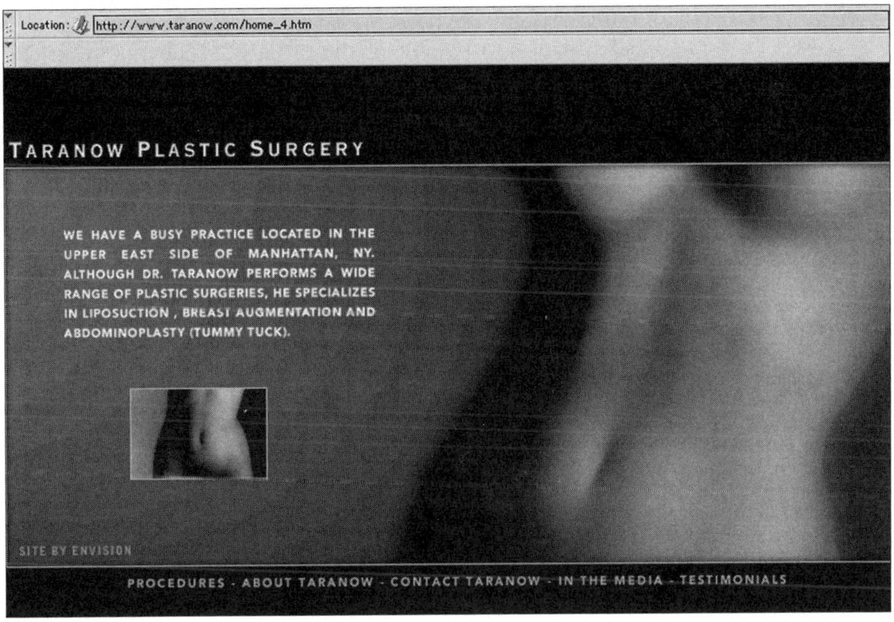

Figure 1.3

The use of the Web to demonstrate outcomes to potential cosmetic surgery patients.

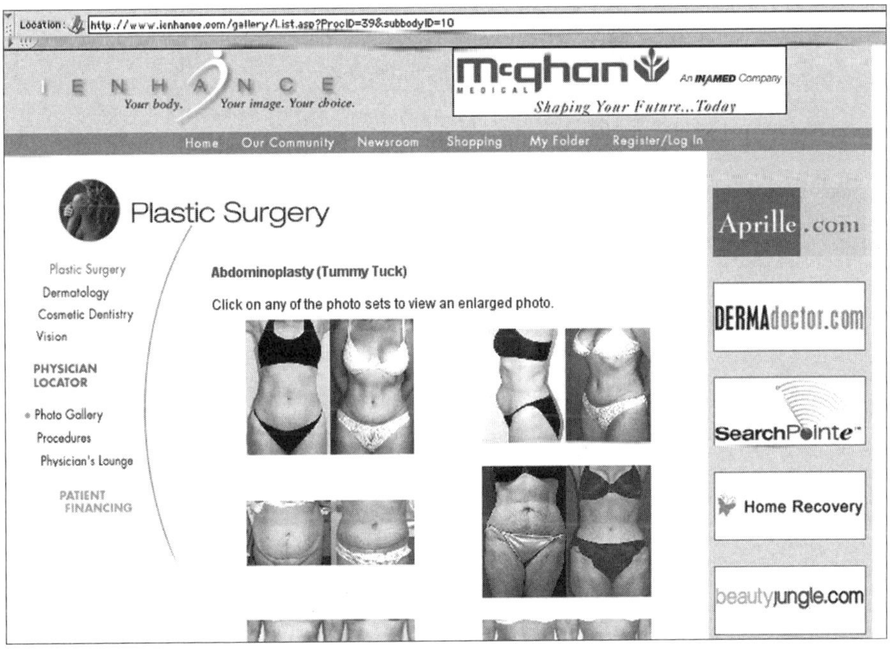

In the following chapters, we cover the basics of marketing as it applies to medical professionals and discuss the specific details of providing an online presence for your practice. At every step, it is important to keep in mind that medicine is different from other businesses, and that an overly aggressive marketing campaign can reflect badly on the perceived professionalism of the practice. However, there is a place for many different levels of advertising in medicine, and some of the most effective and appropriate campaigns are not at all subtle. The billboard shown in Figure 1.4 is a good example of an advertisement trying to appeal to a group of potential patients with a specific need. Presumably, these patients might appreciate a brief, direct message on the road to Las Vegas!

Figure 1.4

Here is a roadside billboard on the outskirts of Las Vegas. This message is simple, memorable, direct, and apparently placed in an area where there may be a significant demand for this procedure.

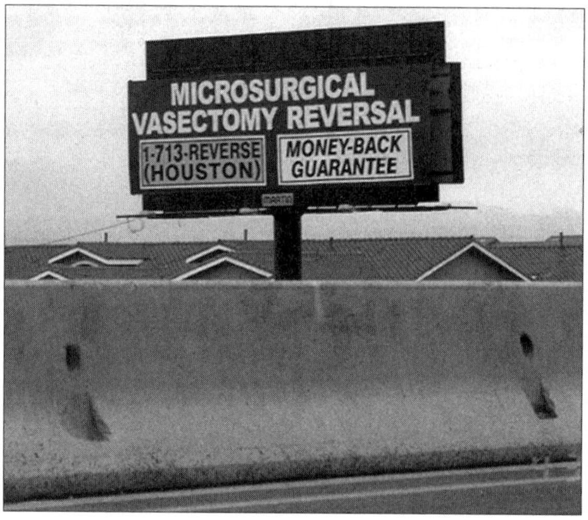

Chapter 2
Early History of the Internet

"With a modem, a phone jack, and an inexpensive computer, your newsroom can be your living room, your bedroom . . . your bathroom, if you're so inclined."

Matt Drudge, Web site creator who first reported the Clinton-Lewinsky story in 1998

Communication

Communication is the necessary foundation of any civilization and culture. It can be as simple as a word or a gesture between individuals, or as rich in form and in content as a classical opera or the entire human genome published on the Internet. While the origins of spoken language are unclear, the medium of written language has been around for the past eight to 10 millennia. Until relatively recently, however, the size of the audience for any type of communication was limited—reproduction of written documents was laboriously slow, and few people could read. Amplification and promulgation of a message primarily depended on the limited circulation of individual text objects or the oral tradition of theater, song, and poetry.

All communication—verbal, written, or symbolic—involves a transmitter and a receiver. The innovation of "mass media" is a greatly increased ratio of receivers to transmitters. Johannes Gutenberg's 15th-century printing press with movable type tremendously enhanced the ability of a single person to send messages to a wide audience. This trend has been exponentially amplified over the past century through radio and television. While broadcast technology has drastically increased the total amount of data provided to the audience, the facilities to publicly transmit information to a large population have, until the advent of the Internet, been prohibitively expensive.

The Internet represents much more than a new way to broadcast information. For the first time, a public medium is truly public in the sense that almost anyone can have access to the transmission end of the broadcast apparatus. Given the right circumstances, an idea originating from a single person can rapidly spread and change the course of world events or affect global markets.[1,2] This represents a quantum leap in human communication that has forever changed many aspects of our culture, such as commerce, socialization, education, political discourse, and entertainment. As we will see in the following chapters, health care is also changing in fundamental ways as patients become more empowered to seek out answers directly and communicate with specialists and other patients around the world.

There are many exhaustive references that outline the development of modern electronic communications,[3,4] and I do not attempt to replicate such a treatment here. Rather, I briefly review the critical events that have led to the modern Internet, for those who are new to this field.

Definitions

Before I start, the definition of a few basic terms may be helpful. (A glossary is also provided at the end of the book for further assistance.)

Two or more computers (or other data processing devices such as printers or scanners) when connected together form a *network*. Such a network has a standard way of communicating, known as a *protocol*. This is analogous to a human language in that if two devices can both "speak" the same protocol, they can communicate if physically connected in an appropriate manner.

Sometimes it is desirable to connect two networks that speak different languages. In this case, some sort of hardware and software are necessary to translate and enable communication between the networks. This translator is known as a *gateway*, and the sum of two connected dissimilar networks is known as an *internet*. (Note the lower case i. Here the term "internet" is generic and applies to any connection between two or more networks.)

There is a protocol known as TCP/IP (Transmission Control Protocol/Internet Protocol), which is the common "language" used for communication between thousands of networks around the world. This massive structure is known as the *Internet* (capitalized). The Internet is one particular instance of an internet that happens to use TCP/IP to communicate. Thus, all of the millions of computers that make up the thousands of networks around the world that are physically connected (through gateways) to the Internet can potentially communicate.

One way to visualize the Internet is as something analogous to the sum total of all the people in the world who speak English. They all have the potential to communicate, given the correct physical connection (such as a telephone line). The analogy goes even further, as many people around the world speak English as a second language. Thus, they have their own internal communications protocol, but have the capacity to connect to the larger global network when needed. Similarly, TCP/IP may not be appropriate for connecting your desktop computer to your printer, for example, so a separate local protocol is necessary. However, it is vital that there be some sort of worldwide standard so that communication is possible between computers (and the people who run them), regardless of their own specific configurations.

Packet Switching and the Creation of the Internet

In 1961, Leonard Kleinrock of the Massachusetts Institute of Technology published a report on the concept of *packet switching*, which is the basis for Internet communications.[5] By this scheme, information (such as an e-mail message, a document, or a Web page) is divided into smaller "packets," each of which contains the source and destination addresses as well as the data to be transmitted. Each packet is sent into the network to be transmitted and reassembled at the other end. The advantage of packet switching is that many users can share a single data line simultaneously, with the various packets taking turns like cars merging into a crowded highway. Furthermore, if there is a transmission error, only a small packet needs to be re-sent, as opposed to the entire file.

DARPA and ARPANET

In 1962, J. C. R. Licklider (also at MIT) suggested the utility of computer networking to further social interactions.[6] Licklider subsequently became the director of the Defense Advanced Research Projects Agency (DARPA), an arm of the Department of Defense. One of Licklider's successors at DARPA was Lawrence Roberts, who had been impressed by this concept of networking. In 1965 (before joining DARPA), Roberts used a standard low-speed telephone line to connect a computer in Massachusetts with one in California, creating the first "wide area" network that did not rely on the physical proximity of its components.

The critical concepts of networking and packet switching were united in September of 1969 to form the earliest version of the Internet. This ARPANET (Advanced Research Projects Agency Network) consisted of two computers at the University of California at Los Angeles (UCLA) and at Stanford (Figure 2.1). One month later, two more computers were added to the project at the University of California at Santa Barbara and the University of Utah (Figure 2.2).

Figure 2.1

Original drawing of the initial two-node ARPANET from September 1969. (Courtesy of The Computer Museum History Center. www.computerhistory.org/exhibits/internet_history/index.page.)

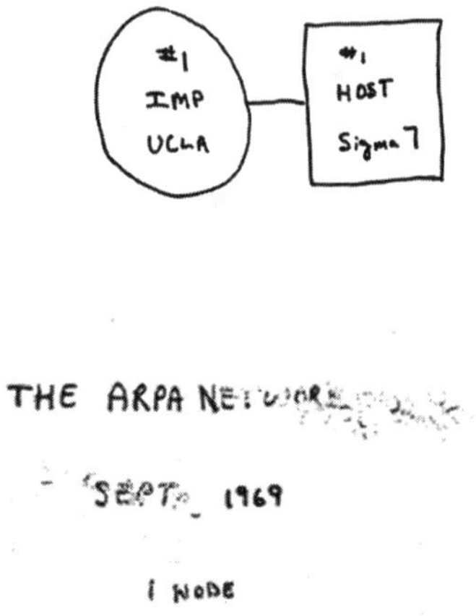

Figure 2.2

Original drawing of the four-node ARPANET from December 1969. (Courtesy of The Computer Museum History Center. www.computerhistory.org/exhibits/internet_history/index.page.)

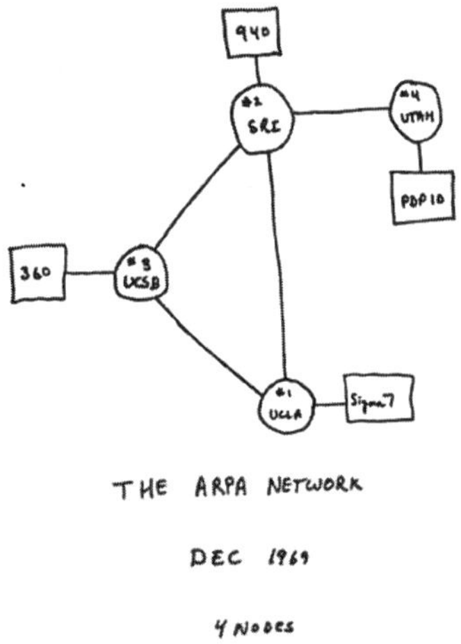

Open Architecture

The next fundamental premise of the Internet was codified by Bob Kahn and Vinton Cerf (among others). Kahn had led the industry team that designed the packet switches for the ARPANET, while Cerf had been on the faculty of UCLA and Stanford. Both joined DARPA in the early years of the Internet, Cerf in 1976 and Kahn in 1972. The critical concept that they developed was that of *open architecture*. This approach maintained that individual network protocols would not be determined by any overall Internet specifications, but that designers of networks would be free to use whatever technology they felt necessary. As long as the network could also deal with a "meta-protocol" that all participating networks would share, communication would be possible.

This meta-protocol was to be born as the previously mentioned TCP/IP. Initially developed for large mainframe computers, TCP/IP software was developed for the variety of desktop computers and operating systems that came into being in the early 1980s. On January 1, 1983, all computers connecting to the Internet were required to transition to this new protocol, replacing the earlier standard, NCP, which had been developed in 1970 for the ARPANET.

Unique Identifiers

The last fundamental Internet concept to be discussed in this chapter is the unique identification required of each individual computer on the network. A computer that is connected directly to the Internet is known as a *host*, and by protocol requirements, each host must have a unique identifying code, or *address*. This address is necessary to label each of the packets of information that flow into and out of it over the network. In the early days of the Internet, the number of hosts was very small, so a single table could be used to keep track of the various addresses. Furthermore, the high-end scientific and military applications that utilized the Internet had no problem referring to these hosts by a numeric code. As the number of individual networks proliferated, and as more and more information consumers needed to access a rapidly expanding number of hosts, the Domain Name System (DNS) was developed (Figure 2.3). This not only allowed for easy-to-remember names to be used in place of numerical codes, but also enabled the table of names and codes to be widely distributed and easily updated across the expanding web of networks that made up the Internet.

Figure 2.3

The growth (in millions) of the number of Internet host computers over the past few years. (Source: Annual July Survey, Internet Software Consortium. www.isc.org.[7])

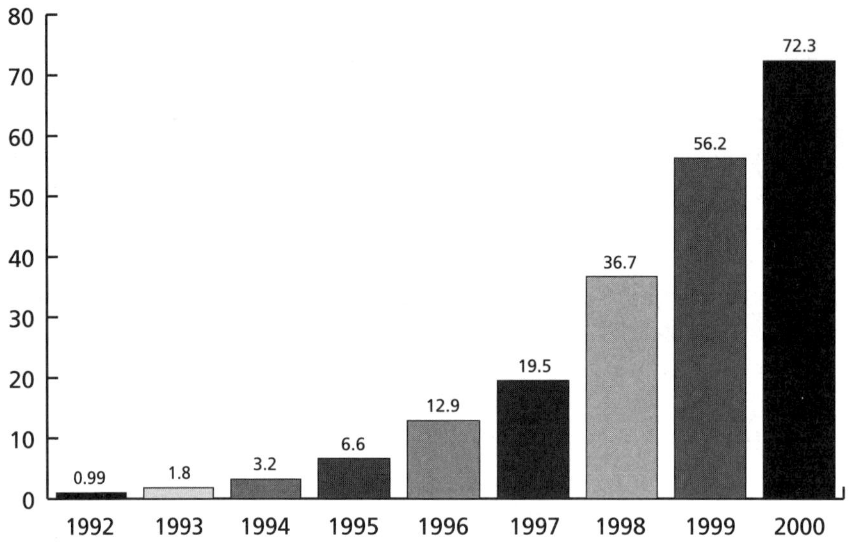

Reviewing the early history of the Internet lets us appreciate how and why its global reach provides us with such a rich and useful communications infrastructure today. In the next chapter, we review some of the basic types of applications that have been developed to take advantage of this infrastructure (such as the World Wide Web). By design, the Internet is a flexible and adaptable system, and new applications are continually being developed.

Endnotes

1. Drudge M. *Drudge Manifesto.* New York, NY: New American Library; 2000.
2. Morgenson G. S.E.C. says teenager had after-school hobby: online stock fraud. *New York Times.* September 21, 2000.
3. Leiner BM, Cerf VG, Clark DD, et al. *A Brief History of the Internet.* Available at: www.isoc.org/internet/history/brief.html.
4. Berners-Lee T, Fischetti M, Dertouzos, M. *Weaving the Web: The Original Design and Ultimate Destiny of the World Wide Web by Its Inventor.* San Francisco, Calif: Harper San Francisco; 1999.
5. Kleinrock L. Information flow in large communication nets. *RLE Quarterly Progress Report.* July 1961.
6. Licklider JCR, Clark W. *On-Line Man Computer Communication.* Cambridge, Mass: Massachusetts Institute of Technology; 1962.
7. Internet Domain Survey. Internet Software Consortium Web site. Available at: www.isc.org/ds.

Chapter 3
Functions of the Internet

"The Internet is like a herd of performing elephants with diarrhea—massive, difficult to re-direct, awe-inspiring, entertaining, and a source of mind-boggling amounts of excrement when you least expect it."

Gene Spafford, Professor of Computer Science, Purdue University

Now that we have briefly covered how the Internet came to be, the functions of this global network of computers must be considered. At a basic level, all Internet applications can be said to fall into one of three broad categories: person-to-person communication (such as e-mail), information broadcasting (such as Web sites), or remote computing. In recent years, these distinctions have become blurred (as in Web-based e-mail) but it is still helpful to think of the functionality of the Internet as falling into one of these broad categories.

Person-to-Person Communication

If the Internet could be summed up in one concept, it would be bringing individuals together through shared information. This global network, beyond the control of any single person or organization, has done more to bridge the gaps between individuals and disparate cultures than any development since movable type. The Internet is intensely personal, in a way that television or literature can never be. Each user has the potential to broadcast and to contact other minds. The first application of the Internet was person-to-person communication, and it remains for many the thing that makes this meta-network so uniquely valuable.

E-Mail

E-mail is often underappreciated. For those who have integrated e-mail into their daily lives, it has taken on an importance close to that of the telephone. While the Web has been hyped extensively and enhanced with ever more complex graphics, sounds, and even video delivery, it still has yet to reach the point where it is deeply integrated into the lives of the average casual Internet user. E-mail, on the other hand, quickly becomes a necessity.

I cannot imagine going a week (or even a day) without responding to my e-mail. Between patient care, academic obligations, and social issues, I find that the great advantage of being able to respond to a problem or a question with a brief comment far outweighs any burden that such an effort might entail. Perhaps you are thinking that I am unusually attached to all things computer-related (and you are right!). My attitude is certainly not yet shared by the majority of my colleagues. However, I believe that a little bit of communication—even while on vacation—can forestall major delays and inconveniences. For example, by having an assistant screen inquiries and subsequently send a daily e-mail with a number of appropriate questions, most problems can be handled with a few seconds of thought, protecting the covering physician. With the right person at the other end screening these requests, some may actually find that a few minutes of online communication makes vacation more relaxing! Of course, this is a matter of personal preference.

E-mail also has the great advantage of extremely low bandwidth requirements. This means that its link to the Internet requires very little in the way of the data-carrying capacity. Contrast this with the Web, which requires a fairly robust Internet connection to even provide simple pictures and will require even more line capacity if it is ever to fulfill the promise of delivering video on demand. You can respond to e-mail messages sent over a pocket pager or cell phone without difficulty, and e-mail has brought the Internet to the developing world where even basic Web service is still not always available.

E-mail can also be used to automatically deliver information. Applications known as *mailing lists* maintain the e-mail addresses of people who sign up by subscribing, signifying their interest in a particular topic. Messages can be sent to the entire group by list administrators (or, in some cases, individual users). This is a convenient way to keep up with a rapidly changing field or an active group with a common interest.

Synchronous Communication

E-mail is a type of *asynchronous communication*, meaning that each message waits for its recipient, and the response is sent at the writer's convenience. There are other communications applications on the Internet, such as Internet relay chat (IRC), that enable *real-time* (*synchronous*) communication through a continuous stream of text. Voice and video communication is also possible, and becoming more and more practical as bandwidth increases. Each mode of communication has its own advantages and disadvantages. Asynchronous communication allows for the (ideally) thoughtful composition of a measured response, with the convenience of responding when and if one is ready. Such communication can also be archived as a meaningful document for future review. Synchronous communication, on the other hand, is more verbal in quality and not intended for archiving (although it certainly can be). This mode is more suited to situations where a rapid exchange of ideas and a dialogue are necessary, such as a conference, a brainstorming session, or a social "chat room."

Information Broadcasting

Over the last few years, the terms *World Wide Web* and *Internet* have become synonymous in common speech. However, the Web is just one particular Internet application developed in 1989 by Tim Berners-Lee and his colleagues at CERN, an international scientific organization based in Switzerland. Originally intended as a method of sharing collaborative documents, because of the popularity and widespread distribution of Web software, many of the other functions of the Internet have been adapted so that they can run through the Web (such as e-mail or file transfers). Nevertheless, the basic function of the Web is the distribution of content (text, images, or other information) through published sites potentially available to anyone with Internet access. There are two key aspects of the World Wide Web that make it such a valuable medium with worldwide reach and infinite expandability: the *generic* nature of the information storage scheme and the possibility of *linking* between resources.

Web Pages, Web Sites, and HTML

A Web *page* is a file containing text written in a language called HTML (hypertext markup language). The important concept of HTML is that this language is a generic way to describe how text and other elements of content (such as sound, animations, images, and so on) should be displayed (Figure 3.1). A Web *site* is simply one or more Web pages residing on a single computer that are connected together (linked) to form a cohesive document, usually built around a common entity or theme.

Figure 3.1

An example of HTML programming in which the generic code on the left is converted into a predictably appearing Web page on the right by a Web browser.

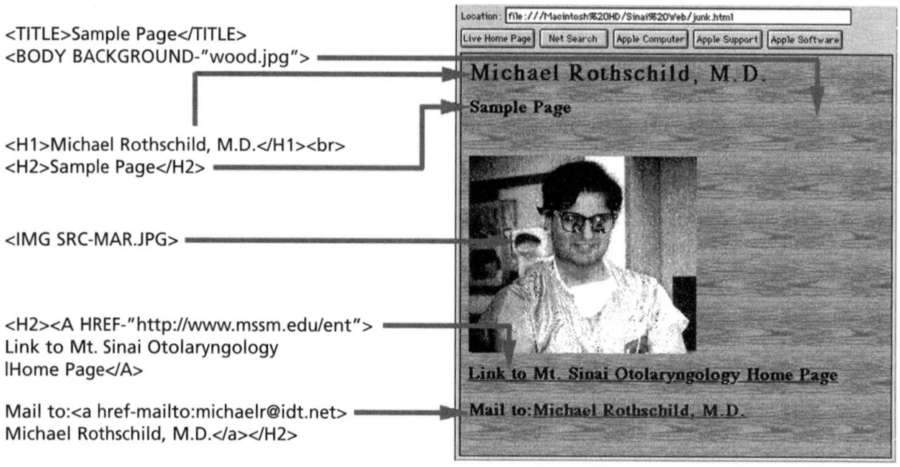

Because HTML is generic, the author can specify how he or she wants the page to look without worrying about what type of computer or software is going to be used to read the page. As long as the reader has a Web browser program, it should be possible to decode the HTML on the page to produce the desired appearance.

Another advantage of using a generic standard language for online resources is that even as the capabilities of computers and other technology evolve, the basic information will still be accessible to the next generation of users. This is clearly important when more permanent data are stored online, such as the archived contents of an academic journal. It is unlikely that whoever is providing such information will continually recode the material to make it accessible as standards change—a time- and resource-intensive project. By sticking to very basic text and image forms, online information can achieve a degree of permanence: perhaps not as much permanence as, for example, the Rosetta stone, but at least more permanence than a document written using a proprietary word processor, which may be practically inaccessible in as little as a decade or so. (For those interested in reading more on the problem of archiving and maintaining works of science and culture in the digital age, I suggest looking at the publications of Stewart Brand, the Getty Conservation Institute, and the Long Now Foundation.[1,2])

Despite its generic nature, as HTML becomes more complex, there are more and more situations in which complicated Web pages will not appear as intended, especially on older browsers. This will be an important thing to remember later on, when you begin making decisions about your Web site design and implementation. A good designer always keeps this point in mind when building a Web site to ensure that the information will be widely accessible and likely to remain so for the near future. Even if sophisticated and elaborate features are used, provisions should be made to allow the informational content to be viewed in some form on simple computers with basic browser software, retaining the advantage of a generic language as described above.

The second aspect of the Web that is a key to its phenomenal utility is the linking of information resources. *Hypertext* is a fairly old concept, even if the term is new—it simply refers to a branching point in a stream of written communication. The simplest example of this is a footnote or reference, where the reader has the option of diverting attention elsewhere temporarily for supplemental related information. Illustrations in a written work are another form of hypertext (*hypermedia*, to be exact, as the supplemental information is nontextual). On the Web, hypertext links enable the author to set the online resource in the context of an ever-expanding and potentially infinite network (or "web") of related information by linking specific points to explanatory text, other Web sites, images, audio, or video elements. Web site construction languages continue to evolve (see the Glossary for definitions of XML, VRML, and DHTML), resulting in improved authoring tools and a richer Web environment.

Usenet

Another type of Internet information broadcasting is found in an application known as *Usenet*. While this application is similar to the Web in that the information is potentially available to everyone with Internet access, it is much more dynamic than the typical Web page that is created and then only occasionally updated. Usenet is a collection of thousands of topic-specific forums known as *newsgroups*. Unlike Web sites, in which information resides on one particular computer and is found by the rest of the Internet community through its unique address, these newsgroups consist of articles of text that are replicated in the many host computers across the Internet. People who are interested in that particular topic will then read the articles posted by other users and respond to the group by posting their own messages (Figure 3.2).

Figure 3.2

A Usenet newsgroup on a medical theme (sci.med.cardiology). These online communities consist of a series of posted messages and discussion threads, often without any assurance or evidence of the qualifications of the author to comment on a particular topic. Nevertheless, the "chatty" quality of the interchanges and the ease with which opinions can be published has made this Internet application quite popular.

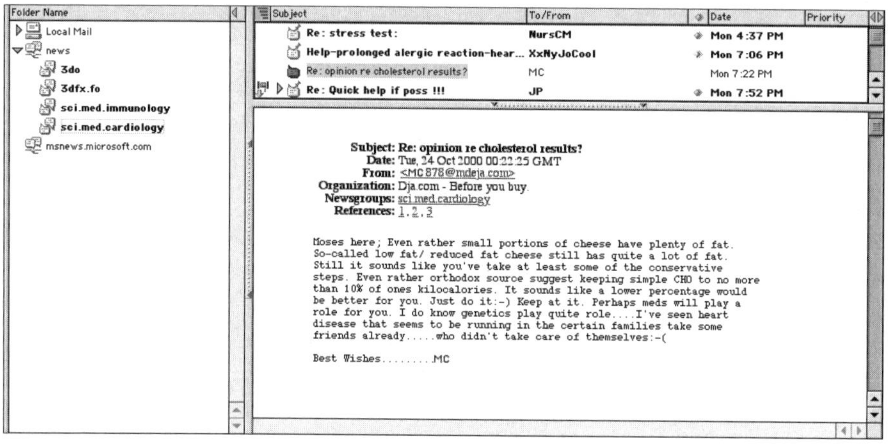

Because there are so many messages posted in the thousands of newsgroups, most Internet hosts only archive a few weeks' worth of recent messages, and perhaps some background files of common interest (such as the "frequently asked questions" documents). The quality of the information in Usenet groups is often questionable, even more so than on Web sites, due to the extreme ease of publishing one's opinion. While these groups can occasionally be useful (as in the exchange of information among support groups), patients must be cautioned about the possibility of erroneous or deliberately misleading information in this venue.

Remote Computing

The last of the three major categories of Internet functionality is remote computing. This implies that the user is performing some task on a computer through an Internet link, as opposed to being in direct physical contact with the computer. Again, the division between remote computing and the last category (information broadcasting) is rapidly blurring, as most remote computing is now done using the Web as a convenient and ubiquitous user interface. However, unlike the usual static Web site, a remote computer is used to perform tasks in real time, dynamically producing Web content that is intended for that specific user at that specific time. Examples of this include the access of online databases, as in the scheduling of air travel, researching the medical literature, or even searching the Web itself for topics of interest (Figure 3.3).

Figure 3.3

Examples of remote computing using a Web-based interface. The user performs database searches on a distant host computer to retrieve airline flight information (A), medical journal references (B), or Web pages on any number of topics (C).

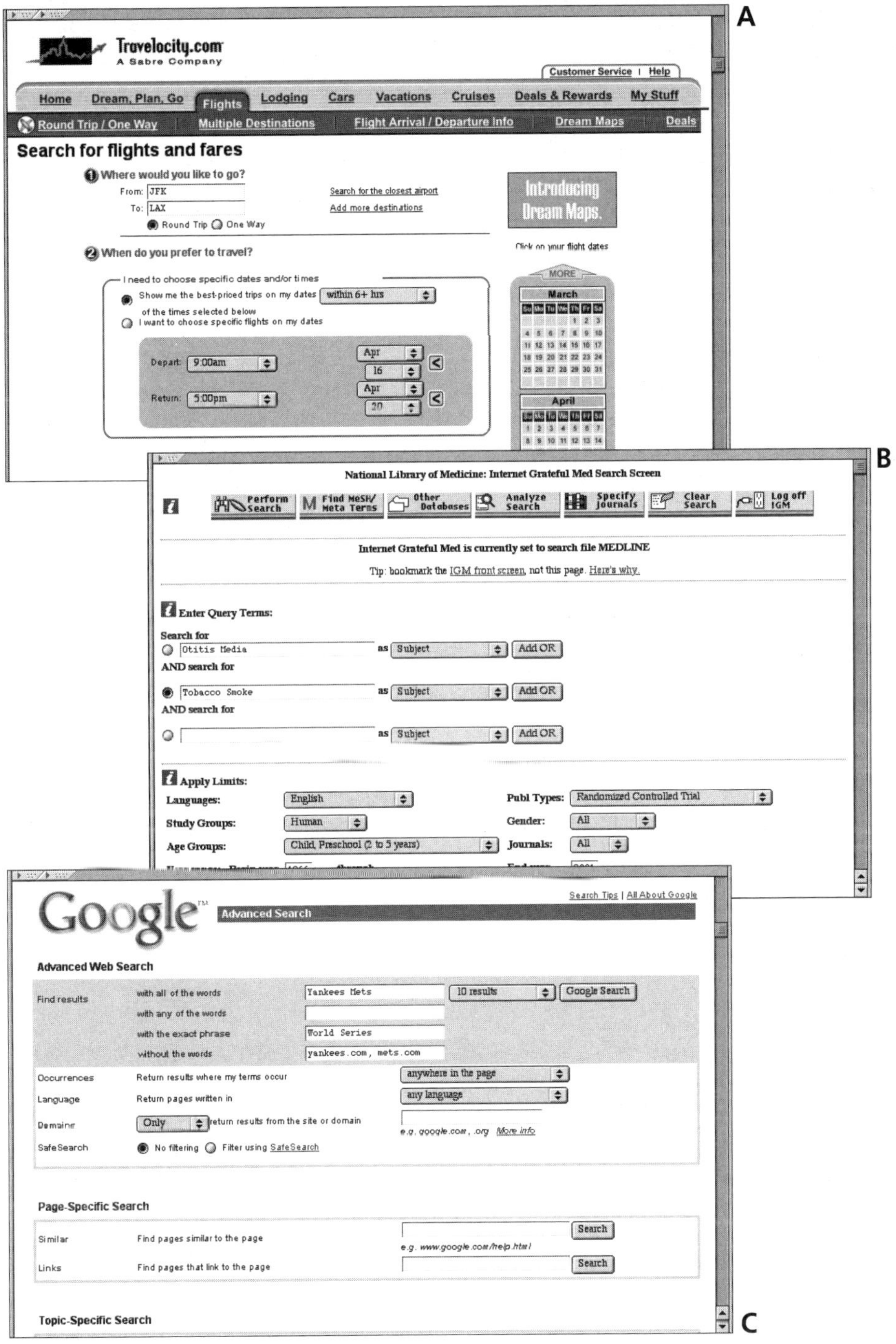

Another example of remote computing that has recently generated interest in the medical community is the "rental" of software through an application service provider (ASP).[3] In this approach, the software is maintained by the ASP on a remote computer, and accessed through the Internet. This is well suited to medical software such as practice management or billing programs. The reason for this is that software purchase prices are typically very high (thousands of dollars) given the relatively small market, and application requirements change rapidly due to evolving federal and state law, as well as changing policies in the managed care industry. By leasing access to software through an ASP, the physician can pay significantly less in the short run, and not be financially tied to a program that may soon be out of date.

Other Internet Applications

Those with significant longtime Internet experience (that is to say, before 1995) may recognize the absence of a number of Internet applications from this discussion. Some of these (such as Telnet, WHOIS, and FTP) remain useful for technically oriented people who work with the Internet at a fairly sophisticated level. Others (such as Archie, VERONICA, JUGHEAD, and WAIS) have been largely subsumed by Web-based applications that fulfill their functions. A complete discussion of such software is available in *A Brief History of the Internet* by Walt Howe.[4]

In the next chapter, we look at how the applications discussed in this chapter have been applied to the field of health care. We also look at how the Internet can be used to support medical decision making, provide clinical information to patients and their families, facilitate the daily operations of medical practices, allow for better communication between health care providers and patients, and help develop "virtual communities" of people with similar conditions. Good marketing of a medical practice must build on these resources to provide something for potential patients besides advertising.

Endnotes

1. MacLean M, Davis BH. *Time & Bits: Managing Digital Continuity.* Los Angeles, Calif: J. Paul Getty Trust; 1998.
2. Brand S. *The Clock of the Long Now: Time and Responsibility: The Ideas Behind the World's Slowest Computer.* New York, NY: Basic Books; 1999.
3. Bazzoli F. Is there an ASP in your future? *Internet Health Care Magazine.* July/August 2000:54-61.
4. Howe W. *A Brief History of the Internet.* Available at: http://www0.delphi.com/navnet/history.html.

Chapter 4
The Medical Internet

"Be careful about reading health books.
You may die of a misprint."

Mark Twain

The Internet is a great tool for patients in many ways, but a caveat is in order. There is widespread belief among patients and their families that the more information one accumulates about a certain condition, the more likely one is to arrive at a correct diagnosis or appropriate intervention. Of course, this is true to a point. The best physicians combine a deep and broad understanding of human biology with an ever-increasing clinical experience and have the common sense to put the two together. Similarly, patients should be educated in the details of their conditions so that they can be intelligent and cooperative partners in care with their doctors.

Too Much Information?

Unfortunately, too much information is sometimes as bad as too little. The lay person attempting to read "everything" about his or her disease may quickly get confused, overwhelmed, or simply misled by the sheer volume of the biomedical literature. Patients can become fixated on one or two articles on an aspect of their illness that may not apply to them. Information published online may lack the most basic scientific validation, and even papers from respected journals may have flawed methodology that has escaped the peer review filter.[1] This was an issue even in the days before the Internet, although the imposing medical library itself served as an impediment to easy research by nonphysicians, and the only writing on most conditions was in scholarly journals.

Since June of 1997, the National Library of Medicine has made its MEDLINE database of biomedical literature available free of charge over the Web through a simple interface.[2] This has made searching the literature quite easy for professionals and the general public alike. Furthermore, the Internet frees would-be authors of health-related information from the traditional limitations of academic publishing.

It can be quite difficult for a patient to distinguish useful resources (such as peer-reviewed science or well-run, disease-specific support groups) from information that is at best untested and ungrounded and, at worst, deliberately misleading or harmful. In the setting of the modern medical Internet, it is the responsibility of the physician to help the patient select appropriate resources and to set them in an understandable context.

The Internet-Savvy Physician

The Internet has revolutionized medicine in many ways, mostly for the better. Patients and doctors alike benefit from enhanced communication, decision support, efficient sharing of medical records, telemedicine, and the creation of online communities in which patients help each other cope with illness. A recent survey by Cyber Dialogue, an Internet-based marketing research company, reported that over 40 million adults in the United States (54% of the population online) use the Web for health information in mid-2000. Furthermore, this number is expected to climb at twice the growth rate of the Internet community in general over the next few years. An estimated 3.7 million adults have reported sending e-mail to a doctor's office, but over 30 million indicated a desire to do so.[3] Of those who expressed such an interest, about 30% claimed they would likely change physicians based on better online access to the practice.[4]

Despite this apparent market for Internet-savvy physicians, the same study also notes that only 4% of online health information consumers are currently interacting with their own doctors' practices online. Although the training of a physician clearly depends on a firm understanding of science, many doctors have limited desire to keep up with technology. Furthermore, unlike many modern businesses, quality medicine can certainly still be practiced without relying on computers—notwithstanding the claims of the most vocal advocates of health care technology.

Finally, most doctors are pressured for time, and have been unlikely to devote significant effort to computer training if they are not already predisposed to do so. Therefore, the acceptance and incorporation of the Internet into the everyday practice of medicine has been far from universal. While a recent study of Web usage in a gastroenterology clinic population suggested that half of the 50% of patients with Web access had recently searched for health information online, only 4% of these patients had ever been referred to the Web by a physician.[5]

Organized medicine has recognized the increasing importance of this new media, and the need to educate physicians about the benefits of incorporating the online world into their professional lives. For example, the American Medical Association (AMA) has provided a number of resources for training doctors in the use of the Internet.[6-8] Although the conventional wisdom has labeled doctors as somewhat "technophobic," this attitude does seem to be giving way as physicians find uses for Internet applications.[9-11] As time goes on, and the Internet is integrated more and more into the delivery of health care, patients will increasingly presume that their physicians are (or should be) familiar with the online world.

Online Health-Related Entities

Fifty years ago, the two main entities involved in the delivery of medical care were doctors and hospitals. This has changed drastically over recent decades—government agencies, managed care, health maintenance organizations (HMOs), preferred provider organizations (PPOs), independent practice associations (IPAs), and large-scale hospital system mergers now populate the landscape with numerous health care entities. Similarly, the Internet contains a wide variety of organizations that are supplying health-related information and services online.

One way of classifying these Internet entities is as providers of the "four C's": content, connectivity, care, and community.[12] (Figures 4.1, 4.2, and 4.3 illustrate examples of Web sites that are focused on one of the four C's.) Content providers supply general medical information, while connectivity providers enable Internet-based transactions between health care entities. Care providers actually dispense specific advice to consumers, and community providers facilitate the association of individuals with common interests, such as disease-specific support groups for patients and their families.

Figure 4.1

An example of a Web site that is focused on content.

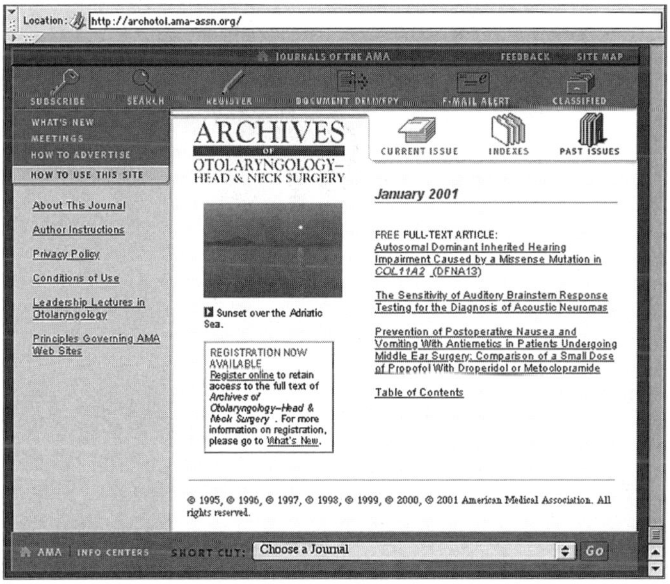

Figure 4.2

An example of a Web site that is focused on care.

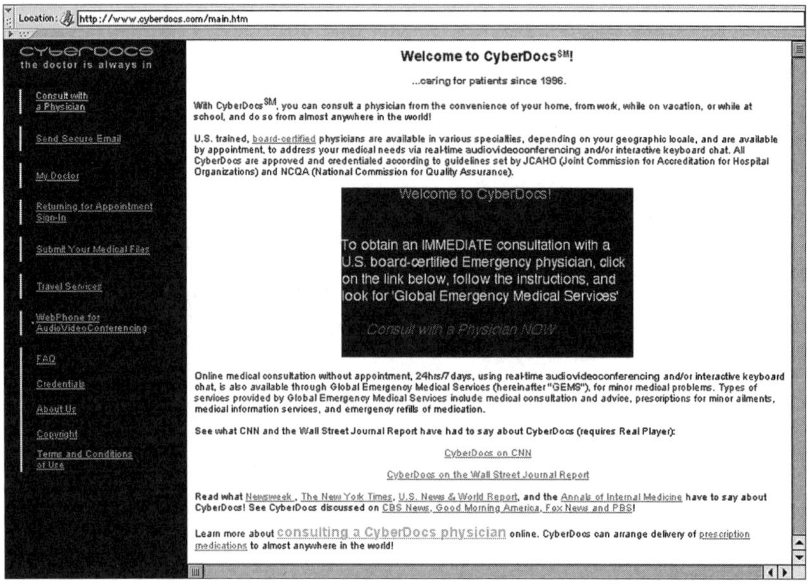

Figure 4.3

An example of a Web site that is focused on community.

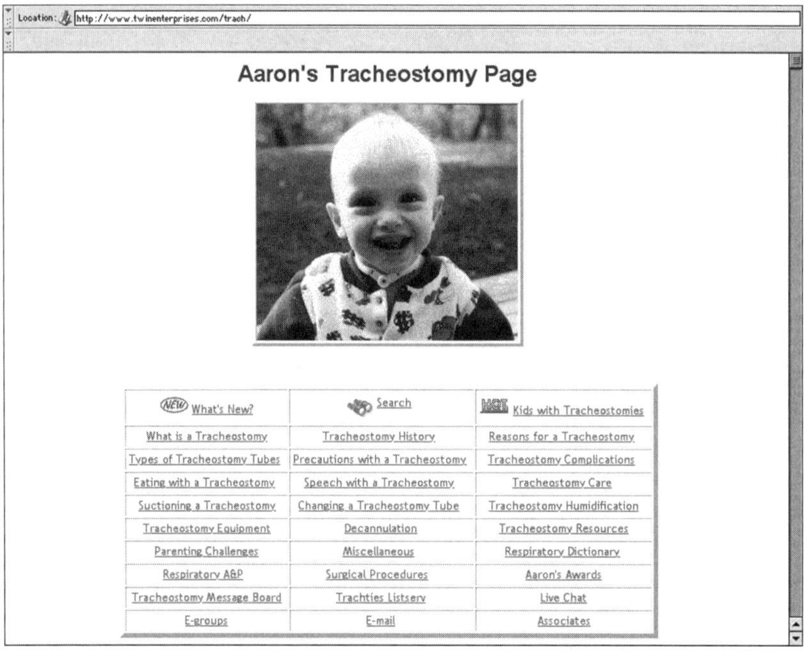

Supplemental Information Broadcasting

Over the past 2 years, I have run a simple Web site (www.Kids-ENT.com) to provide information about frequently encountered conditions in pediatric otolaryngology. In the course of this time, the site has generated nearly 2000 e-mail exchanges with patients around the world. In corresponding with many of these individuals, I have confirmed my suspicion that there is a major communications gap between doctors and patients. Many of these correspondents are frustrated by their inability to get answers from their local treating physicians.[13]

This gap is not necessarily from lack of care or compassion on the part of the doctor. The clinical encounter is usually stressful for the patient and family members, and all of the best-intended teaching may go unheard, especially if the news is bad. Frequently, doctors lapse into technical language and patients are not inclined to press for further clarifications. Not every doctor is skilled at communication, and misunderstanding may occur despite his or her best efforts.

The Internet is well suited for supplementing the discussion that occurs in the consulting room. A Web site can be custom made by the physician to cover the specific approach that reflects his or her practice preferences for any situation. It is available 24 hours a day, and can be reviewed as needed by the patient. A Web site is much easier to keep up to date than printed brochures, and it can be accessed by the patient from anywhere in the world. A good Web site can take the place of a 3 AM phone call after surgery when the typical postoperative course is outlined in detail. Furthermore, specific practice details can be easily included such as directions to the office (complete with maps generated from any starting point), insurance participation, office hours, credentials, and new or unique procedures available through the practice.

Web sites are an excellent way of providing static information to patients. Sometimes, however, they do not cover a specific situation or further clarification is needed. By providing a means to contact the physician or other office staff members on a nonemergent basis, e-mail can be far superior to the "telephone-tag" that many patients play with their doctors before getting through. Furthermore, all such communication is automatically documented, and can be printed out for inclusion in the office chart. As long as it is clear when to use e-mail and when to use the telephone in case of an emergency, the Internet can be a tremendously valuable asset to a busy practice. (This topic is discussed in detail in Chapter 10.)

Internet Journals

Information broadcasting on the medical Internet takes a number of forms. Usenet newsgroups enable people with similar interests to "publish" their opinions in a global (if transient) forum. Vast numbers of Web sites have been generated on health-related topics, by physicians and other health care providers, as well as by patients, insurance companies, pharmaceutical companies, and other entities with an interest in this field. Traditional medical publishing has also moved to the Internet, as established print journals migrate their content to the Web. New Web-only journals are seeking to establish a reputation and attract original peer-reviewed research for online publication.

The difficulty of publishing medical information in the past was a function of the cost of the media and the limited space available in established biomedical journals. This limitation was a good thing in many ways, as it served as a check valve on the prodigious output of the world's authors. Although far from perfect, the system favored scientifically valid research that passed peer review. The reader was assured of the quality of the published information by the reputation and authority of the editorial staff.

To be sure, politics has always been a part of academics, and over the years good science has been denied publication for reasons unrelated to intrinsic merit. However, with the advent of Internet publishing, the floodgates have truly been opened. It is now our responsibility as physicians to guide our patients as they search for information online and help them learn how to determine which information is good and which is incomplete, misleading, out of context, or even nefariously published for material gain.

Numerous start-up companies have endeavored to create medical Web portals that act as clearing houses and filters for online information, but from the patient's viewpoint, this task is far from complete. Even the most respected "brand names" can have problems with conflicts of interest, especially when questions arise regarding the flow of advertising revenue that maintains the site.[14] This has been a problem since the first advertisement appeared in a medical journal, and editorial independence has been fiercely protected by academic publishers throughout the years. Hopefully, similar firewalls between scholarship and business will be maintained as medical publishing enters the Internet age.

The legal, ethical, and academic issues of medical publishing on the Web have been extensively discussed in recent years.[15-19] However, those physicians who provide original medical content through the Internet would be well served to consider some of the suggested guidelines for appropriate health care information broadcasting before posting a personal opinion for the world to read. (These guidelines are discussed further in Chapter 9.)

The Online Medical Record

Many physicians practice in geographically separated offices or accept telephone calls at home from patients after hours. Furthermore, traveling patients may require medical care while away from their regular physicians and their medical charts. Additionally, in an emergency room situation, the treating physician rarely has access to a well-documented past medical record. It is potentially unsafe to make medical decisions without all of the appropriate data, yet this has been the *de facto* standard of care for years. If the patient's chart were accessible through the Internet, his or her entire medical history could be read from anywhere that had Web access (eg, doctors' homes, hospitals, or multiple medical offices). Several companies have begun to provide this service in the form of a personalized home page with password-protected, patient-specific information tied to a medical chart (see Figure 4.4).[20,21]

Figure 4.4

An example of a pediatric practice Web site that provides secure personalized accounts for parents, enabling them to access their children's medical records through the Internet.

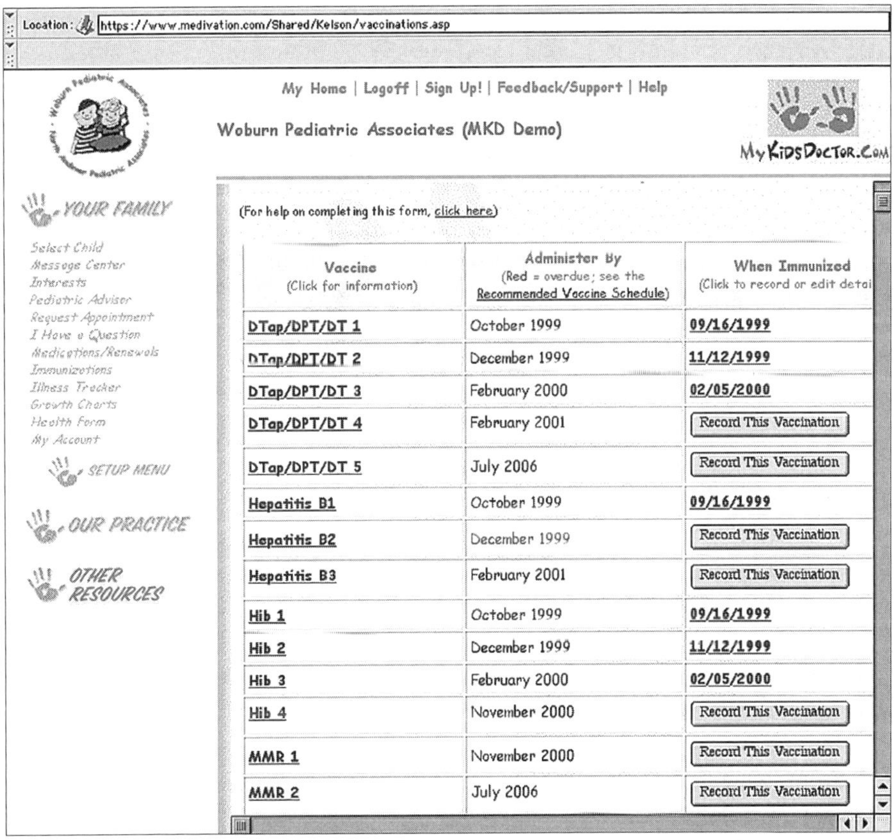

Privacy Concerns and Legislation

Although accessing patient records online is an appealing prospect, there are tremendous concerns regarding the security and privacy of online data, and these need to be addressed before the Internet becomes a standard repository for the patient chart. A full discussion of this topic is beyond the scope of this volume, as patient-specific records have yet to become a standard feature of medical practice Web sites. However, a few "cutting edge" practices have indeed allowed patients to maintain secure accounts within their Web sites, through which limited portions of the medical records are accessible. At this writing, however, such personal health records have not been widely instituted and data storage and retrieval protocols have not been standardized.

Another reason for the delay in the widespread adoption of Internet-based patient records in the United States has to do with upcoming federal legislation. In 1996, the United States Congress passed a law known as the Health Insurance Portability and Accountability Act (HIPAA). This act was intended to help patients who were changing employers to maintain their health care coverage, and to facilitate the transfer of health records from one employer or care provider to another. The effect of this law is that the federal government will establish standards for all entities engaged in the electronic transmission of health care information, covering privacy, security, transactions, code sets, and identification numbers for health care providers, consumers, and clearinghouses.

Over the past 4 years, several hundred thousand public comments have been considered in the course of codifying these regulations. The first set of rules based on this legislation was published in the *Federal Register* on August 17, 2000, and a sweeping implementation of the HIPAA privacy regulations was issued a few months later in December 2000. Although the complete codification of these rules will not be completed for some time, compliance is mandated by October 2002 (October 2003 for smaller care providers such as individual doctors' offices).

While it is not clear at present exactly how these regulations will be implemented and enforced, it is surely vital that any new software involving the online access of health records be made HIPAA-compliant as the law is implemented. The recently issued privacy regulations are particularly controversial. Critics claim that full compliance may paralyze health care delivery, while privacy advocates state that they are necessary to protect patient's interests as medical information is increasingly handled through electronic data interchange. As of this writing, it is not clear whether the incoming administration will reduce this administrative burden to give relief to the health care industry, or support the rule in its current form. Some analysts predict that the cost of HIPAA compliance may be more than twice that spent by the same companies for Y2K compliance. (For further information on this important topic, see the full text of the law or one of the many articles written on HIPAA and its impact on the health care industry.[22-25])

A Caveat

As we have seen, the Internet is poised to revolutionize the practice of medicine in many ways. However, doctors can be quite the traditionalists, both in their clinical practices and in their approaches to information management. The "cutting edge" of online health care gets a lot of coverage in the media. Early adopters of technology have embraced and publicized applications such as telemedicine, Internet-based medical records, claim submission through the Web, and even the online auctioning of medical procedures![26] While many of these applications may at some point become mainstream, the vast majority of physicians still use pen and paper for their chart notes. Most doctors will continue to insist on seeing a patient face to face before offering a diagnosis or suggesting a procedure. Many desirable features of the medical Internet still are impractical or incompletely implemented due to technical limitations and lagging health care policy initiatives.[27] There is a tremendous amount of inertia both at the institutional level and at the individual practitioner level—in some ways this is a good thing. Eventually, standards will develop and online health information systems will be sufficiently stable, flexible, and scalable to allow for widespread adoption. However, we are not there yet.

Endnotes

1. Biermann JS, Golladay GJ, Greenfield ML, Baker LH. Evaluation of cancer information on the Internet [see comments]. *Cancer.* 1999;86:381-390.
2. Internet Grateful Med. National Library of Medicine Web site. Available at: http://igm.nlm.nih.gov/.
3. Cyber Dialogue releases Cybercitizen Health 2000. Cyber Dialogue Web site. Available at: www.cyberdialogue.com/news/releases/2000/08-22-cch-launch.html.
4. Cyber Dialogue reports that doctors are missing internet health opportunity. Cyber Dialogue Web site. Available at: www.cyberdialogue.com/news/releases/1999/10-12-cch-doctors.html.
5. O'Connor JB, Johanson JF. Use of the web for medical information by a gastroenterology clinic population [in process citation]. *JAMA.* 2000;284:1962-1964.
6. Chi-Lum BI, Lundberg GD, Silberg WM. Physicians accessing the internet, the PAI project: an educational initiative [editorial]. *JAMA.* 1996;275:1361-1362.
7. Internet Health Road Show. American Medical Association. Available at: www.ama-assn.org/about/roadshow/index.htm.
8. Bryson DM, Ingebretsen M. *The Physician's Guide to Internet Explorer: A Quick-Start Tutorial.* Chicago, Ill: American Medical Association; 1999.
9. Barrett MJ. *The Forrester Report: Why Doctors Hate the Net.* Available at: www.forrester.com/ER/Research/Report/0,1338,9114,FF.html.
10. Stevens L. Still having growing pains. *Medicine on the Net.* 2000;6:1-4.
11. Chin T. In search of the killer app. *American Medical News.* 2000;October 9:31-32.
12. Gruen J. The physician and the internet: observer or participant? [published erratum appears in *MD Comput.* 2000 Jan-Feb;17(1):12]. *MD Comput.* 1999;16:46-48.
13. Eysenbach G, Diepgen TL. Patients looking for information on the internet and seeking tele-advice: motivation, expectations, and misconceptions as expressed in e-mails sent to physicians [see comments]. *Arch Dermatol.* 1999;135:151-156.

14. Noble HB. E-MEDICINE—a special report: hailed as a surgeon general, Koop is faulted on web ethic. *New York Times.* September 15, 1999.
15. De Ville KA. Internet listservers and pediatrics: newly emerging legal and clinical practice issues. *Pediatrics.* 1996;98:453-454.
16. Elliott SJ, Elliott RG. Internet listservers and pediatrics: newly emerging legal and clinical practice issues. *Pediatrics.* 1996;97:399-400.
17. LaPorte RE, Marler E, Akazawa S, et al. The death of biomedical journals. *BMJ.* 1995;6991:1387-1390.
18. LaPorte RE, Hibbitts B, Smith R, Horton R, Lundberg GD, Davidoff F. Rights, wrongs and journals in the age of cyberspace. *BMJ.* 1996;313:1609-1612.
19. Rothschild MA. Otolaryngology and the internet: e-mail and the world wide web. *Otolaryngol Clin North Am.* 1998;31:255-276.
20. Logican/MedicaLogic Web site. Available at: www.medicalogic.com.
21. My Kid's Doctor Web site. Available at: www.mykidsdoctor.com.
22. HIPAA Administrative Simplification. Department of Health and Human Services Web site. Available at: http://aspe.hhs.gov/admnsimp.
23. Goedert J. The dawn of HIPAA. *Health Data Management.* April 2000:84.
24. Bazzoli F. Keeping data safe. *Internet Health Care.* September 2000:56-63.
25. Pear R. New privacy rules are challenged. *New York Times.* December 21, 2000.
26. Bid for Surgery. MedicineOnline.com Web site. Available at: www.medicineonline.com/bid4surgery.
27. Amatayakul M. The NRC report. Is healthcare ready for the internet? [in process citation]. *MD Comput.* 2000;17:47-48.

Chapter 5
Internet Marketing and the Marketing of Medical Practices Online

"A few years ago not a single commercial had an Internet address. How many advertisements today exist without one? Half of them? And within two years there won't be any left."

Bill Gates, April 2000

While advertising is frequently the tool that builds a modest business into a tremendous success, most enterprises have a fairly limited advertising budget. In order to get the most productivity out of invested dollars, a decision must be made as to where these funds should be allocated. As little as 5 years ago the idea of Internet marketing may have been laughable to many companies; however, the phenomenal growth of the online audience and the relative economy of the media have made the Web (and even e-mail) a standard part of the advertising budget today.

Advertising Trends

Reviewing recent trends in the advertising industry helps demonstrate the rise of Internet marketing. Over the past few years, the majority of the approximately $200 billion spent annually on advertising in the United States went to the "Big 3" media: television, newspapers, and direct mail (Figure 5.1). Internet advertising makes up a fairly small portion of this pie, only about $4.6 billion in 1999. While accounting for under 3% of the total dollars spent, Internet advertising represents about twice the amount spent on outdoor advertising (eg, billboards), and has more than doubled since 1998. The growth trend continues, as spending on Internet advertising in the first quarter of 2000 was equal to the 1999 total![1,2]

Figure 5.1

Distribution of the $172 billion spent on advertising in 1999 (United States).

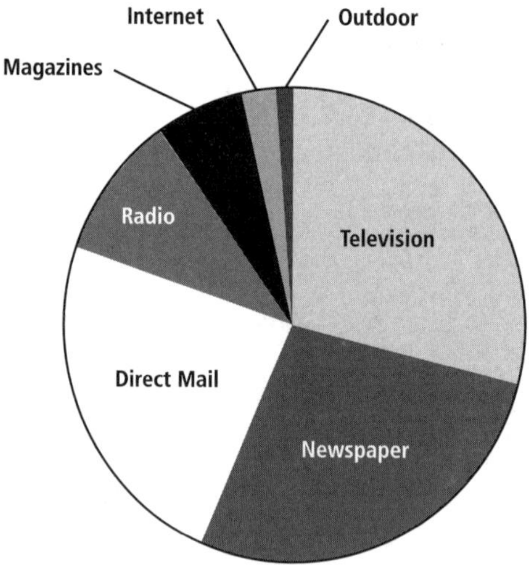

These numbers, however, do not fully explain the meteoric rise of Internet advertising. Advertising space—on television, in a newspaper, or on the Internet—is priced as CPM, or *cost per thousand* viewer impressions. (The "M" refers to the Roman numeral representing 1000.) CPM for Internet advertising space is significantly lower than that of traditional advertising, and dropping. The intrinsically lower cost of producing Internet advertisements (as compared to, for example, television ads) means that the actual product exposure per dollar spent is potentially much higher. As one contributor to an online marketing journal put it: "At current CPM levels it would be possible to buy about four times the number of impressions you can get on TV, billboards, etc, and know for sure that people have the immediate ability to click through."[3]

If CPM were the whole story, however, no one would ever advertise on more expensive media such as television. Of course, the bottom line in any advertising venture has to be the generation of revenue through sales (leaving aside public service advertising or political advertising, whose efficacy is measured in behavior modification). For commercial advertising, which is the model we consider here, the outcome of interest will have to be another advertising metric, the CPS, or *cost per sale.*

Consider an example taken from a Forrester Research survey. A Web site advertisement (often called a "banner ad") has a CPM of $16, meaning that it costs the advertiser $16 for every 1000 people who view it. The *CTR* (click-through rate, or the percentage of people who will click on the ad to learn more) is about 0.8%, and the conversion rate (the percentage of those people who buy the product) is

2%. Therefore, the total CPS is \$100 (16 / [1000 × 0.008 × .002]) A direct-mail marketing campaign, on the other hand, has a CPM of \$850, which seems very high. On the other hand, we all get a lot of direct mail, so it must be cost-effective! The reason is that the conversion rate is actually quite high (1.2%), and the click-through rate is not really applicable, as the conversion rate reflects those who don't even open the envelope as well as those who look at the ad but do not buy. The CPS for this direct-mail campaign is actually \$71, lower than that for the Web site banner ad.[4]

Of course, this is something of an oversimplification for illustrative purposes. Some people might buy through other channels after being exposed to either of these advertisements, and if the goal is to build global name recognition on a limited budget, the low CPM might offset the relatively higher CPS. While placing banner ads on high-volume Web sites (such as Yahoo!) can provide global publicity at a fairly low CPM, it can also be quite expensive as the total cost is proportional to the CPM times the number of site visitors (the Internet equivalent of a television commercial aired during the Super Bowl). The cheapest form of online advertising is viral marketing, in which an online "buzz" is created about a product through e-mail lists, newsgroups, chat rooms, and the like. When enough people are convinced that the product is valuable, the message propagates on its own (like a virus), with high efficacy and essentially no cost. The appropriate type of advertising depends largely on the product or service being marketed, as we will now consider.

Types of Businesses

For the purpose of this discussion, there are three types of businesses. The first is a traditional business, run from one specific location (although a single company may control thousands of individual franchises). A product or service is provided to individuals who are in physical proximity to the business location. This type of business is called "brick and mortar" by the Internet community—an image that captures both the good and bad aspects of physical permanence in a specific location. Doubling the customer traffic of such a business generally entails an attendant rise in all costs, such as raw materials, consultation time, or administrative staff (although there may be some economies of scale and the marginal cost of servicing the last customer may be fairly low). Typical examples include restaurants, retail stores, and medical practices.

The second type of business also provides a physical product or service that is delivered to individual clients, but without the need for physical proximity. A central location receives orders and ships product, but the "selling" is done remotely (eg, by telephone or on the Internet). The potential customer base is huge, limited only by the physical means of delivery. Doubling the customer traffic still entails an increase in material costs and processing staff, but there need not be an increase in the cost of receiving and tracking the orders if this is done automatically through the Web. Examples of this include online bookstores or catalog-based retail outlets. The company itself can be an extension of a physical store ("click and mortar") or solely distribute products or services through online sales ("Internet pure play").

The third type of business exists only online. The product or service is "virtual" and the potential customer base is the entire online community. The entire transaction, from marketing the product to taking orders, filling them, and billing the customer, is done through the Internet. Apart from the (dropping) price of bandwidth, doubling customer traffic would double the gross revenues with no increase in expenses. The marginal cost of servicing the next customer is essentially zero, and the business is thus considered to be extremely "scalable." Examples of this type of business are Internet portals and search engines.

Marketing Considerations

There is overlap between these three categories of business, especially in the area of marketing. A local brick and mortar business, such as a franchised restaurant, will benefit from a national advertising effort for the chain, whether online or through conventional media. A catalog merchant may depend on a local showroom but also take telephone orders as well as orders through a Web site. Indeed, the more "virtual" some aspects of the business can be, the better. A sale made through a catalog merchant's Web site will have a lower overhead cost than the same sale made through a telephone operator or by mail order.

When considering how to market a medical practice, it may seem less than efficient to spend extensively on Internet promotion. After all, medicine is very much a brick and mortar business, and the vast majority of people who are exposed to your advertisement are unlikely to be potential customers. Unless you are running an internationally renowned tertiary care center or are a physician who provides a service unavailable anywhere else in the world, your patient base is generally local. Widely distributed advertising (such as a banner ad on a major portal) is likely to be wasted; directed marketing is better for a medical practice, which has a target audience limited by geography and their need for health care.

Despite these considerations, however, there are considerable advantages to online marketing for medical practices. As mentioned previously, the cost should be fairly low to develop a Web site, and ongoing maintenance costs should be negligible. For certain types of practices, a single new patient obtained through the Internet might offset the costs of the online presence for years. A practice Web site need not be advertised solely online (eg, through banner ads), but rather by offline promotion (such as business cards and letterheads), directed toward referring physicians and patients. The site can also be promoted through the manipulation of the various search engines and directories, which will cause the site to be referenced when searches are done based on a particular condition (see Chapter 12).

An online presence brands a medical practice as being current in its application of technology, as well as being interested in enhancing communication between doctors and patients. Certainly, at this point, most of the senior clinicians and national leaders in patient care and research completed their training (and much of their careers) in a world without the mass-market Internet. It would be wrong for the public to assume that the lack of a major online presence implies less than first-rate health care. However, over the next few years, Web sites and e-mail accessibility may become the norm rather than the exception for medical practices. In this setting, the lack of a Web site or online access may be considered a significant omission by prospective patients, similar to the lack of an after-hours phone answering service.

While not directly affecting patient flow, the Internet may also allow for increased profitability by assisting with cost- and resource-intensive processes, such as patient registration, record keeping and distribution, laboratory follow-up, call-backs, and even billing. In addition to identifiable savings, such efforts can make the practice run more efficiently, translating into better patient satisfaction, retention, and new referrals. This enhanced efficiency is definitely a marketable aspect of the practice, which will distinguish your services from less patient-friendly competitors. As mentioned previously, however, these applications have not been widely implemented and may be subject to a variety of industry and federal regulations in the coming years.

Any Web site based on a medical practice is a type of "advertising." Traditional marketing of physicians has centered on the generation and maintenance of a good reputation through training credentials, successful outcomes, a strong work ethic, and good communication skills. This is summarized in the "three A's" of medical practice—affability, availability, and ability (note the traditional order of the terms!). The online presence of a medical practice is not the typical direct sales effort that characterizes commercial advertising. Rather, it promotes the practice by building "brand recognition," by providing a useful resource for health-related information, and by demonstrating the practice's emphasis on good doctor-patient communication.

Traditional advertising does have a place in medicine, but less so in the promotion of an independent clinical practice. Just as hospitals have begun to buy more and more air time for commercials on radio and television, health care providers may advertise through ad placement on high-volume, health-related Web portals or even through unsolicited e-mail. It must be remembered, however, that this type of marketing has a much higher CPM (and CPS) than a freestanding Web site, in which the costs are essentially fixed no matter how many people visit the site.

The Integrated Marketing Strategy

The goals of marketing any product or service are well established. More recently, the integrated approach to marketing has become popular. This concept is simple: marketing should be part of a synchronized effort in which a variety of media and channels are used to convey the same message. From the standpoint of marketing a medical practice, this means that whatever particular value your practice provides to the community should be linked to recognizable public images (eg, a logo, health care philosophy, specialization profile, and so on). This public image should appear to the extent possible on your Web site, your letterhead, your business cards, and any publicity items that promote your name in the community.

The Goals of Marketing

1. *Educate the target population about your product or service.*
2. *Distinguish yourself from the competition.*
3. *Cut through the background noise with a simple, memorable message delivered at the appropriate time and place to a receptive audience.*

To begin planning an integrated marketing strategy, a realistic assessment of the communities' needs is vital, as discussed in Chapter 1. Next, specific marketing goals should be outlined and the appropriate target audience identified. The most common goal is typically the generation of consistent revenues, especially in the early years of a medical practice. In the business world, this is traditionally divided into the capture of new customers and the continued patronage of established customers. The latter should not be neglected, as satisfied patients are often the best source of new referrals.

It can be quite difficult to attract new patients, as medicine in most communities is essentially a "zero-sum game." Apart from people moving into an area, or families who have just had their first child, most new patients are lost from other practices. In addition to dissatisfied patients, this group includes those who need highly specialized services not available within the referral network of their own primary care providers, or those who are forced to switch practices for insurance reasons.

Once the public image of the practice has been characterized, the main goal of integrated marketing should be to display this image to the community of potential patients in as many forms as possible. If the practice is a regional center of excellence, this should be highlighted on a Web site, in the local news media, in the yellow pages, and anywhere else appropriate. The practice logo should be not only on envelopes, letterhead, and business cards, but also a prominent feature of the online presence (see Figure 5.2). Conversely, the Web address should be displayed on all printed materials.

Figure 5.2

The incorporation of the same practice logo into more than one information channel, using an integrated marketing approach. The practice has in this way reinforced the message provided by the Web site (A), the newsletter (B), and the return mailing address on envelopes (C). (Courtesy of the Heart Institute of Spokane.)

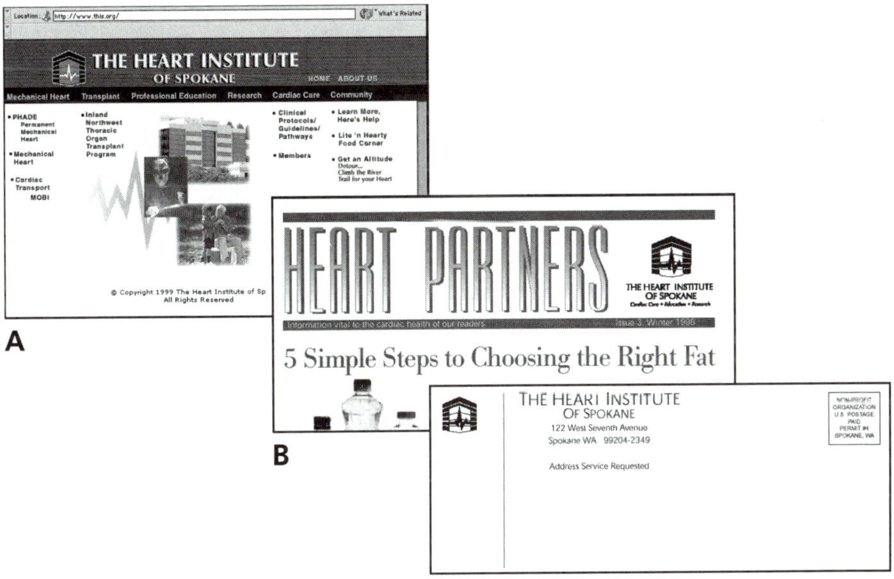

A

B

C

By following the integrated approach, not only will each marketing effort reinforce the others, but content produced for one medium will be available for use elsewhere without duplicating work. Personal profiles of staff members, electronic CVs, photographs, practice philosophy statements, and graphic design elements can be included everywhere from billboards to Web sites to brochures.

Endnotes

1. Universal McCann-Erickson U.S. advertising volume. Advertising Age Web site. Available at: http://adage.com/dataplace/archives/dp446.html.
2. Internet Advertising Bureau Web site. Available at: www.iab.net.
3. Tchong M. Issue: Can a "dotcom" company succeed with an online-only ad campaign? Iconocast Web site. Available at: www.iconocast.com/issue/1999102103.html.
4. Forrester Research. The big E: e-mail dispatch. Iconocast Web site. Available at: www.iconocast.com/issue/2000021703.html.

Chapter 6

Creating an Online Presence: The Budget and the Approach

"A billion here, a billion there, and pretty soon you're talking about real money."

Senator Everett Dirksen

Now that a comprehensive plan has been developed for an integrated marketing effort, the realities of the budget must be applied. As a nonscalable business, there is a limit to the productivity of each physician. Herculean marketing efforts and extensive spending on promotion of a medical practice may actually backfire, resulting in more work than can be handled by existing staff. In times of managed care, negotiated fee reductions, and capitation, even expanding the number of providers may not be cost-effective for an individual practice. Therefore, the marketing budget must be developed in the context of the current level of services and the potential for handling new patients from the community.

It Takes Money to Make Money

As was mentioned in Chapter 5, spending on Internet advertising is rapidly growing, and exceeded $4.5 billion last year in the United States. At the same time, revenues of medical practices are trending downward as managed care matures and more and more clinicians are moving toward negotiated discounted fees or capitation. Funds are scarce for all practice expenditures, and budget items must be carefully considered. However, the old adage "it takes money to make money" applies in this situation—without good practice development, the best medical training and skill are wasted.

Many traditional businesses allocate approximately 8% of their revenues for marketing, and expect a return on this investment of 300% or more to justify the effort. As noted previously, it may be difficult to accurately track the efficacy of an advertising budget, as new business comes from a variety of sources, and multiple motivating factors may be at work to produce a new customer or to close a sale.

In the field of medicine, the situation is even more complex, as different patients may provide different returns for the same successful marketing effort (depending on insurance status). Furthermore, overly aggressive marketing may negatively impact on a practice's perceived reputation, resulting in lost business that is never noticed or accurately attributed.

In conventional business, Jay Levinson's theory of "guerrilla marketing" suggests that there are three groups of target customers.[1] The first target group is every possible customer in the business' potential geographic reach (which may be the entire world for Internet businesses). The second target group is a subset of prospects who are considered to be more likely to respond to a marketing effort. The third target group consists of established customers, in hopes of repeat business. This approach to marketing suggests that the budget be broken down to allocate 10% to the first group, 30% to the second group, and 60% to the third group. The theory here is that the greater the potential for a "sale," the higher the return on the advertising investment.

Medicine, again, is different from most businesses. While you would certainly like your patients to return to your practice if they need health care services again, we do not generally think about approaching our established patients to encourage further utilization of services. This may be the effect, however, of a dedicated program of health education and the encouragement of preventive medicine (such as cancer screening, cardiovascular monitoring, dental checkups, and so on). In this regard, continued contact with patients who are not in a state of acute health crisis is a type of marketing to the third group, and can result in better public health as well as fuller utilization of practice resources. Do not neglect to promote your online presence to your established patients as a source of education and possibly a channel for continuing communication with you and your office staff.

Creating a Medical Practice Web Site

There are three basic approaches to Web site creation, and an initial decision must be made as to which of these will be most appropriate for your practice. Creation of the site may be outsourced completely to a Web design company. Alternately, the site can be created automatically by a "wizard"—an online program provided by a sponsoring organization that will quickly construct a personal practice site based on the answers given to a series of questions. Finally, the option remains of doing the project yourself. There are advantages and disadvantages of each of these approaches, which we will now explore.

Outsourcing to an Internet Professional

Outsourcing to a design company may be the best choice for most practices. If a concerted effort is to be made to market your practice online and enlarge your referral base through the Internet, I do not recommend skimping on the online marketing budget. Web designers, public relations experts, and graphic artists are professionals, and deserve to be well reimbursed for good work. While it is true that you can draw your own practice logo and put together a Web site with minimal training or talent, your online presence reflects on your practice. In the days of the early Web, almost any site was considered interesting by the few people who had the capacity to view it. Today, however, people have become sophisticated in their surfing, and a "homemade" Web site reflects poorly on the professionalism of the practice it represents (Figure 6.1).

Figure 6.1

An early medical Web site, circa 1995 (A), and a professionally done modern Web site (B).

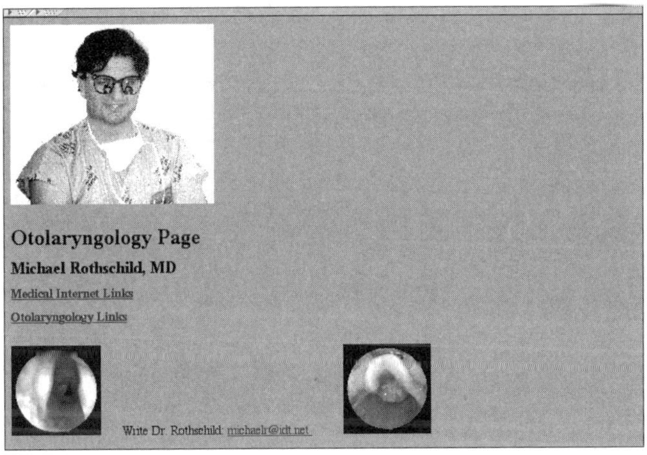

A

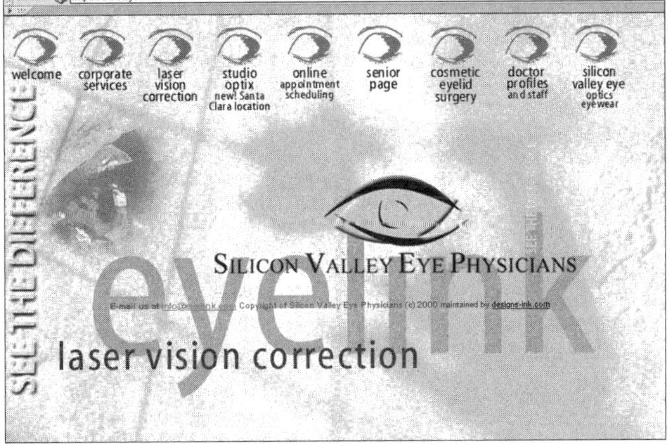

B

With this last point in mind, be prepared to spend several thousand dollars if you want a unique Web site designed around your practice. Many professional Web design companies have appeared over the past few years, some offering a full suite of services in addition to Web page creation (such as market research, site promotion, or interactivity with patients). It is important that the firm you choose have significant experience working with medical practices. In some cases, a national medical society will partner with a Web design firm to provide customized sites with access to proprietary medical content.[2] This arrangement usually involves a significant discount to members as well as an ongoing relationship with the sponsoring group.

Be sure that you fully understand what is and what is not covered in a design firm's quoted price, and understand that there will be (smaller) ongoing costs as well (Figure 6.2). Also be sure to reserve some portion of your marketing budget for promotion of the Web site itself. While Web services can represent a significant cost center for many large businesses, an individual medical practice should not be spending much more than $5000 on assembling a handcrafted, individual site. Indeed, as more and more Internet marketing firms are launched, competition has driven down prices considerably, as has the advent of free site-building wizards by several large medical entities such as Medem (sponsored by the American Medical Association and several other national medical societies), Salu.net, or Medscape.[3-5]

Figure 6.2

Costs associated with developing an online presence. Initial costs typically consist of marketing consultation, graphic design, Web site design, and assistance with content development. Ongoing costs usually consist of hosting, promotion, and content maintenance fees.

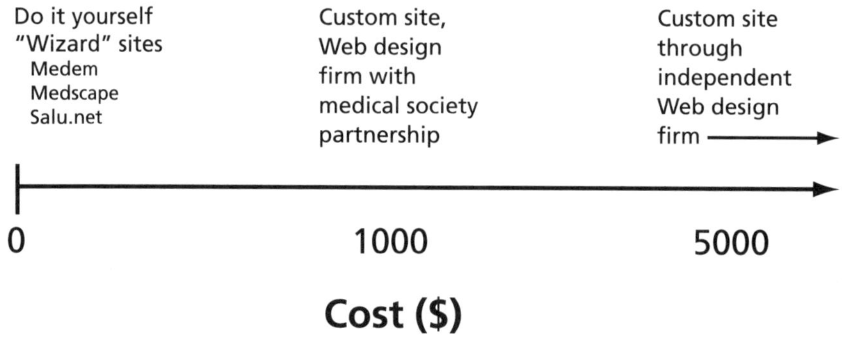

Automated Web Site Creation

Wizard-produced Web sites tend to be similar in appearance and have fairly limited potential for customization. However, for many practices, using a Web site wizard may be more than adequate for providing basic information to existing patients or to new patients referred through conventional means. If there is no great need to aggressively market the practice online, this approach can be a useful and economical alternative. Furthermore, many of the organizations providing free Web sites can also supply extensive collections of content available for posting on individual practice pages. For example, Medem has copyright access to informational materials provided by its member organizations, which at this writing include the AMA, nine other national medical societies, and two state medical societies. Doctors creating Web sites through this service can pick from a library of archived articles on a variety of specialties for inclusion on their informational pages. Furthermore, frequently updated news feeds can add current content to the pages automatically.

One disadvantage of the wizard approach is the lack of ownership of a unique domain name (Web site address). Each of these services provides an address for your site that is linked to its own Web servers. It is always possible that the terms of service under which your site was created can be changed in the future, as the domain and the site itself remain the property of the sponsoring organization. Furthermore, the marketing advantage of an easily remembered domain name (discussed in Chapter 11) is somewhat diluted by attachment to the domain of the sponsoring entity (see Table 6.1). Again, for many practices, this may not be a tremendous disadvantage, but it should be considered before much effort is put into promoting the Web site—the domain name will need to be widely reproduced on business cards, letterheads, and other printed materials. Finally, the wizard approach provides the least customization potential, giving the site an "off-the-rack" look, which may be less than optimal for marketing purposes.

Table 6.1

Addresses Used for the Kids-ENT Web Site, With Domain Names Registered Independently or as Subdomains on an Organizational Server

INDEPENDENT	www.Kids-ENT.com
MEDEM	www.Kids-ENT.yourmd.com
MEDSCAPE	http://doctor.medscape.com/Kids-ENT
SALU.NET	www.Kids-ENT.salu.net

Doing It Yourself

The third approach to site creation is "do it yourself." For all but a very few physicians, this is probably the worst choice. One of the most frequent questions asked by doctors considering an online presence is, "What kind of software should you use to create a Web site?" This is something like asking what brand of word processor is best for writing a novel. The answer is that anyone can write a novel with any sort of word processor, but to write a *good* novel, you need to be a talented writer! The important questions should be: "Why do you want to create your own site from scratch, and are you really capable of doing it well?" Two or three years ago there weren't a lot of other acceptable options. As of this writing, however, it is fairly hard to justify such an effort, given the rising expectations of the Internet community for professional look and feel, as well as the falling costs of producing either a professional customized site or a wizard-generated site.

For those few physicians with the time and the talent to justify a Web-authoring project, there are a wide variety of tools available for the job.[6,7] HTML editors range from simple text editors up to sophisticated WYSIWYG ("what you see is what you get") software packages. Some provide facilities for rapid uploading to the Internet and for online editing. Furthermore, there are a number of Web sites that will automatically grade your site by checking the page loading rate, the status of the links, its compatibility with various browsers, and other features, such as Netscape's Web Site Garage Web page and Doctor HTML's Imagiware Web site.[8,9]

The bottom line, however, is that most physicians are not interested in Web authoring—they are interested in having a Web site. Unless you have a good artistic sense and truly enjoy working with computers on a fairly basic level, primary Web authoring is probably not time well spent. You will likely find yourself spending large amounts of time and effort to develop an online presence that is not as well designed as a professional customized site, nor has as much content as a site produced under the aegis of a national medical organization.

Web Site Funding

Finally, let us consider the tempting idea of funding the Web site through Internet-based revenue streams. It may be appealing to try to defray some of the costs of a Web site through strategies such as banner ads or corporate sponsorship. A banner ad is simply an advertisement designed to fit in a small strip (banner) on a Web page. The owner of the page is paid a certain amount to display the advertisement, just as a landowner might be paid for billboard space. Furthermore, these banner ads are interactive, in the sense that clicking on the banner will take the viewer to another Web page (presumably one belonging to the advertiser). Extra payment to the host page may be negotiated for each such visit, known as a "click-through." Alternatively, a company might sponsor an entire Web site—underwriting the costs of development and maintenance—in return for labeling of the site with the sponsor's name. Some pharmaceutical companies have done this for a variety of medical Web sites.

Such revenue-producing ventures are rarely justified on Web sites of individual medical practices. Even the most elaborate, custom-designed site for an individual practice should be relatively inexpensive when compared to the potential return on the investment. Furthermore, even the most successful of such sites is unlikely to attract the level of Web traffic needed to make advertising space valuable. Banner ads consume bandwidth and slow down the page loading rate, making any Web page less appealing.

More important, however, is the impact that advertising or direct sponsorship can have on the public impression that the site makes in the Internet community. Trust is perhaps the most important commodity in the medical Internet. If visitors get the impression that a conflict of interest exists, or that the site is on some level an advertisement for a particular drug, the perceived value of the site will be severely reduced. It is not difficult to find an example of how even a limited conflict of interest can overcome a reputation for impeccable ethical standards.[10]

Budget for your online presence like you would for any other practice essential. Given the range of options available, it should not be difficult to fund a useful Web site out of any practice's operating expenses. Just as you wouldn't display an advertisement or the name of a drug company on your car, resist the temptation of "something for nothing." There is always a catch!

Endnotes

1. Levinson J. Guerrilla Marketing Web site. Available at: www.gmarketing.com.
2. ENTLink Web site. Available at: www.entlink.net.
3. Your Practice Online. Medem Web site. Available at: www.yourpracticeonline.com/Medem/html/splash.html.
4. Salu Web site. Available at: www.salu.net.
5. Medscape's Free Physician Web Pages. Medscape Web site. Available at: www.medscape.com/medscape/homepages.
6. Dekker F, St John D. *HTML for Beginners.* CNET Web site. Available at: www.builder.com/Authoring/Basics.
7. Musciano C, Kennedy B. *HTML & XHTML: The Definitive Guide.* Beijing: O'Reilly; 2000.
8. Web Site Garage Web page. Netscape Web site. Available at: http://websitegarage.netscape.com.
9. Doctor HTML Web page. Imagiware Web site. Available at: http://drhtml.imagiware.com.
10. Noble HB. E-MEDICINE—A special report: Hailed as a surgeon general, Koop is faulted on web ethic. *New York Times*. September 5, 1999.

Chapter 7
The Look and Feel of an Effective Web Site

"...it is a tale told by an idiot, full of sound and fury, signifying nothing."

William Shakespeare, Macbeth

This book is in no way meant to be a primer on Web authoring—there are numerous superb online and printed tutorials covering the subject in depth.[1-3] Therefore, I do not go into detail regarding such topics as table creation, form incorporation, Java scripting, or the implementation of image maps. However, as there are so many ways to make a site virtually useless through the overuse, or misuse, of the many features available to Web authors, I feel that a brief discussion of design issues is appropriate at this point. Any doctor who establishes a customized online presence should have some familiarity with Web design to be an intelligent partner with the site's Webmaster.

There are three major aspects of any Web site that contribute to its overall quality and the efficacy of communication: the site's "look and feel," its internal linkages, and its external linkages. The "look and feel" of the site refers to such things as the choice of color combinations, background textures, text styling, layout, and elaborate features such as music, animation, or interactivity. *Internal linkage* refers to the way the individual pages of the site form a cohesive whole. *External linkage* refers to the points in the site where reference is made to resources elsewhere on the Internet. In this chapter, we discuss issues of a site's look and feel; in the next chapter, we explore issues related to internal and external linking.

As any marketing executive will tell you, look and feel is an extremely important concept. Major lawsuits have turned on the issue of how closely one product resembles another. While most of us do not have the talent to produce great-looking documents, billboards, or television commercials, we are an extremely sophisticated audience for these forms of expression. Having grown up marinating in a sea of media, we readily notice subtle differences in type font, color combinations, or the layout of elements on a page. Advertising agencies spend millions of dollars on psychological research to determine which elements are effective and which are not, which evoke positive feelings toward a product or service, and which are jarring or unpleasant.

With this in mind, be sure that any Web designer you hire either has significant experience in this field, or utilizes the services of an appropriate graphic artist. It is critical to examine sites created by any potential consultant for these qualities, and your own instincts may be your best guide.

It is difficult to simply list the elements that make up an appealing Web site. Efficacy and visual appeal arise from a cohesive whole, and there is no simple formula for success. On the other hand, it is quite easy to identify features that are less than desirable. Thus, good design can be taught by looking at bad examples. The classic Web authoring text, *Web Pages That Suck: Learn Good Design by Looking at Bad Design* by Vincent Flanders and Michael Willis, takes this approach.[1] Let us now consider some of the basic elements of a Web site and typical pitfalls that can reduce the site's quality.

Layout: Text, Blank Space, and Frames

Layout refers to the arrangement of text and graphics on a page. A confusing layout is one of the first mistakes made by the novice Web author. Because there is an inclination to include as much information as possible on the very first page, it is easy to allow the layout to become distracting and unfocused. Blank areas of the page can be effective if used with artistic understanding. However, too much blank space makes the site look unfinished and lacking in content, while too little blank space reduces readability and causes the main points to be lost in excess verbiage.

Frames are a feature of some Web sites that enable a browser to display several windows simultaneously. This can sometimes be helpful in controlling the layout of the site as viewed by the visitor. Frames can also allow for the display of material from other Web sites without actually sending the site visitor to that site. This approach keeps the visitor at the original site while displaying outside resources in a separate window (Figure 7.1).

Figure 7.1

The use of frames to display outside resources while maintaining control of the visitor's browser. (A) Material from the Kids-ENT.com Web site is displayed in a frame within the main Kids-ENT.com site. (B) An outside resource (the JAMA home page) is displayed within the frame on the Kids-ENT.com page. Note that the user has not actually left the Kids-ENT.com Web site to view this material.

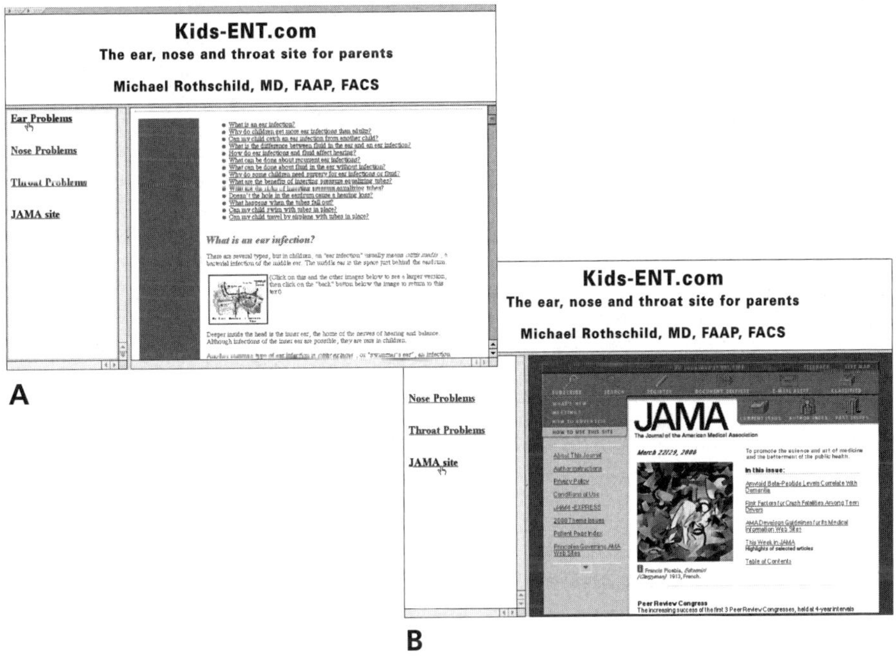

Unfortunately, some older browsers have difficulty displaying frames correctly, and even if they display as intended, it can be confusing for the user to face multiple scroll bars when attempting to view the contents of each window. Furthermore, screen real estate is a valuable commodity, and dividing it up into small packages with space-eating scroll bars can impair the overall utility of the page (Figure 7.2). Frame usage may also interfere with indexing by search engines, reducing the likelihood that the site will be found. A frame page is difficult to bookmark and may cause problems such as crashing of the browser. For these and other reasons, frames should be used sparingly, if at all.

Figure 7.2

An example of the overuse of frames.

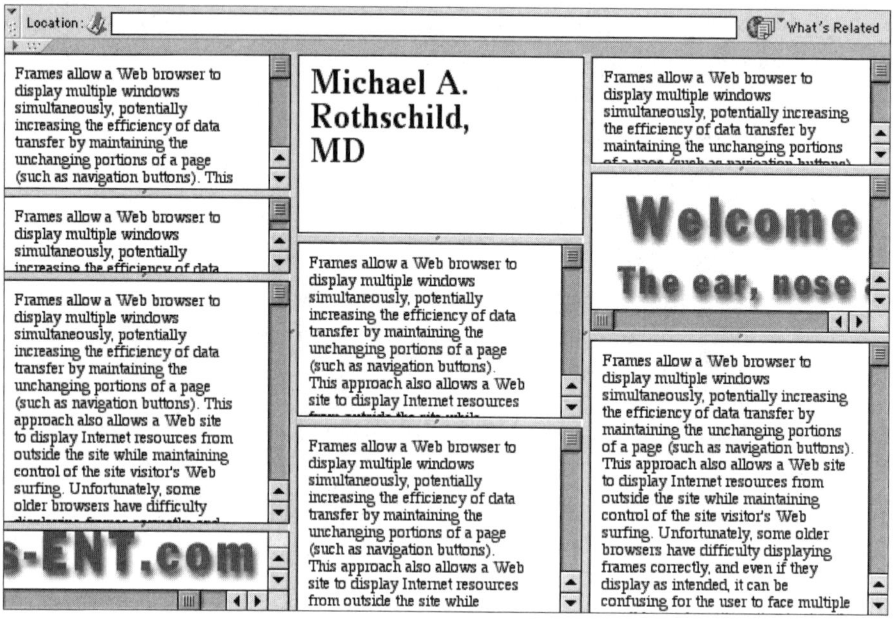

Designing for the Lowest Common Denominator

Although HTML is meant to be generic, resulting in the same appearance on any computer, the truth is that there are subtle differences in the way various computers and browsers interpret a given Web page. This is more evident as the site becomes increasingly sophisticated and complex, incorporating new features of the Web that may not be fully implemented in every browser. For this reason, it is important to make sure that the pages appear as desired in multiple settings, including at least the three major browsers (Netscape's Communicator, Microsoft's Internet Explorer, and the America Online browser). The arrival of new browsers as well as the proliferation of Web-enabled electronic devices such as handheld organizers and cellular phones only complicate things further. If you are expecting your site to be viewed in a variety of settings, it might be best to provide an alternative text-oriented site with minimal graphics but similar content. Remember, when designing the overall layout of a page, consider the lowest common denominator. Many pages look great on large, high-resolution monitors, but not every potential site visitor has such hardware.

Colors and Textures

Jarring combinations of colors can make a Web site quite unpleasant. While this may be intentional in certain artistic settings, such a design should be avoided on medical sites. Furthermore, insufficient contrast between the background color and the text, or between the colors used for text, links, and visited links, can make navigation difficult. There is simply no substitute for good design.

The incorporation of background textures is always tempting. Because these files are very small (and cover the entire page by being tiled, or displayed multiple times), they take up little bandwidth and do not appreciably increase the page loading rate. And, to be fair, they can be effective and evocative, giving, for example, the impression of a marble countertop or a wooden bench. Unfortunately, backgrounds can be distracting and take away from the text unless they are extremely subtle or the text consists of only a few, large words (Figure 7.3). A detailed background is usually not the best choice for a content-heavy medical Web site.

Figure 7.3

Distracting background textures impair the readability of a Web site.

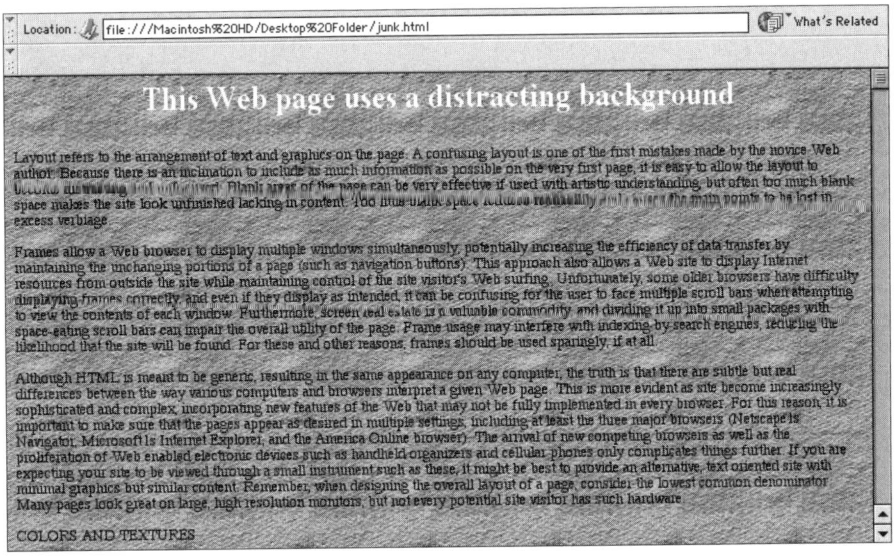

One of the few Web standards is the set of colors that identify links. Text that serves as a link should be identified by the standard blue color, which then changes to purple after the link is visited. (This scheme helps users keep track of where they have been on a page with a lot of links.) Links are traditionally underlined as well. Using any color scheme other than this may make for some confusion, especially among those new to the Web. Furthermore, using underlining for nonlinked text is also confusing and should be avoided if possible.

Fonts and Styles

The fonts used for text passages should be plain and unembellished. Flourishes—such as the extra lines in the so-called "serif" fonts—can make reading from a monitor more difficult. The clean lines of the sans-serif fonts typically make for better readability. Furthermore, a font that is likely to be available on a wide variety of computers should be selected; otherwise, substitution will occur and the final appearance may not be as intended by the designer. Fonts that are generally available on Macintosh computers and those running the Windows operating system include Arial, Helvetica, Times, Times New Roman, Courier, and Courier New (Figure 7.4). Arial and Helvetica are sans-serif fonts and are quite popular online. Times and Times New Roman are serif fonts and are commonly found in print. The courier fonts have the appearance of typewritten text, and are occasionally used to add a "retro" touch to selected portions of a Web site.

Figure 7.4

Fonts commonly available for use in the display of Web sites.

Arial
Helvetica
Times
Times New Roman
Courier
Courier New

Text style refers to text attributes such as boldface, italics, underlining, and the weight or size of the letters. The judicious use of these styles will result in a page that looks professional and directs the reader appropriately. The excessive use of such features makes the page seem confusing and illegible. For example, the "blink" style makes the text blink on and off on the screen. In the early days of Web design, this was considered extremely sophisticated, as any sort of motion on a Web site was rare. Today, however, blinking text is considered to be poor form and should only be used rarely (if ever) to draw attention to a specific word (such as "New!").

Style sheets are a method of incorporating multiple stylistic specifications into one HTML command. This has the advantage of allowing global changes in appearance without extensive rewriting of the basic code. This is good, as most Web sites go through many iterations before an acceptable version is achieved for public display. Style sheets also allow for rapid reworking of the basic page layout.

Images

The average Web user has very little patience for pages that are slow to load. If the site is not visible in a few seconds, many people will leave before seeing any content at all. While other network factors can cause slow downloading, the most common cause of this problem is the use of graphic elements that are too large or overly detailed. Even though more and more people are using high-speed Internet connections, the majority of consumers still reach the Web on relatively slow dial-up modems, making slow page loading a continuing problem.

There are a number of ways to minimize this delay when preparing images for online viewing. First, only include those images that are truly necessary. Not every piece of screen real estate needs to be covered with unique graphics. Second, minimize the file size of those graphics that you do include. When creating these images, remember that screen resolution is 72 dots per inch (DPI). Any image with a higher level of detail will likely still be displayed at 72 DPI, but expanded to larger physical dimensions, requiring scrolling and wasting bandwidth.

While 72 DPI seems low when compared to printed images that can be 150 to 300 DPI or more, it is actually more than adequate for most Web site images. This is because a computer display automatically enhances the perceived level of detail. The pixels (tiny points of color that make up the picture) are actively emitting light from a CRT monitor or laptop LCD screen. Thus, 72-DPI images appear much sharper onscreen than they would if printed at this resolution, as a print is only visualized through the ambient light it reflects.

Most online graphics are stored as either GIFs (graphics interchange format) or JPEGs (Joint Photographic Expert Group format). These are methods of compressing image files so as to take up less space online. In general, JPEG is optimal for photographs, while GIFs are better suited to artwork, drawings, and other images with less complex edges and a smaller number of different colors. The newer PNG format (portable network graphics) may soon become the standard for online images, as it is superior in many ways to GIF, which it was designed to replace. Among other advantages related to compression algorithms, PNG is free for public use (unlike the GIF format, which is proprietary software).

The GIF format saves space by reducing the total number of choices in the color palette (the range of possible colors for display). The number of unique colors that can be displayed in any image depends on the number of bits of information the computer assigns to each pixel. (This is also called *color depth.*) Eight bits (that is, eight ones or zeros) allows for the description of 256 different numbers, and therefore 256 different colors for each pixel. Dropping to 7 bits reduces the number of colors to 128, but this may not actually be very noticeable. By the time the color depth is reduced to 3 bits, only eight colors are available. A 3-bit palette results in degradation of quality if the image contains any subtle shading of tone (Figure 7.5). If, on the other hand, the image has only a few contrasting colors (such as a flag or a cartoon), no degradation would be visually detected (Figure 7.6).

Figure 7.5

A continuous-tone (photographic) image, compressed using the popular JPEG, GIF, and PNG formats. A magnified view is included for each image, to emphasize the different types of image degradation obtained with each compression scheme. The original image (A) was scanned at 300 DPI, 409 × 261 pixels, full color, and was approximately 5.3 MB in size. In the GIF format image (B), the palette has been reduced to 3 bits (8 colors), resulting in a significant savings in terms of file size (180 KB), but the image quality suffers. Note the "posterization" effect of a limited color range (the lack of smooth transition between adjacent areas). The JPEG version (C) was saved at low quality. The file is only 120 KB in size, but the fine detail is lost. Note how the picture breaks up into "granules" when viewed at higher magnification. The image quality of the PNG file (D) is excellent, although the file size savings using this format are not as great (900 KB). Remember that the quality options on the GIF and JPEG files shown here for comparison have purposely been set extremely low to demonstrate image degradation. The actual file size difference between PNG, GIF, and JPEG for comparable quality images is not as pronounced, and is usually indistinguishable when viewed on a monitor at the appropriate resolution and size.[4-6]

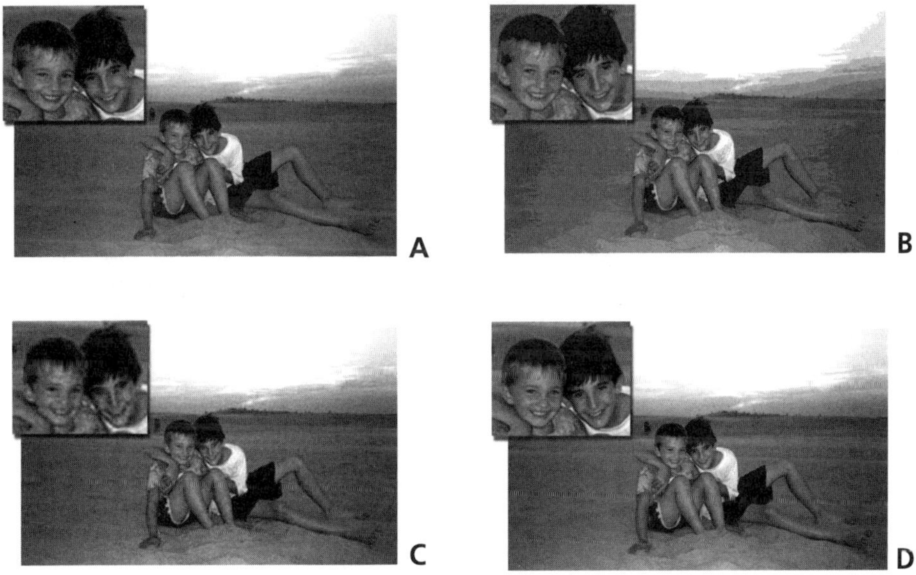

Figure 7.6

A simple three-color drawing. The appearance is identical whether displayed as the original image, or compressed using GIF, JPEG, or PNG formats. The original image was 29 KB in size, the low-quality JPEG version was 25 KB, the PNG version was 18 KB, and the GIF image using 3-bit color depth (8 colors) was only 9 KB in size.

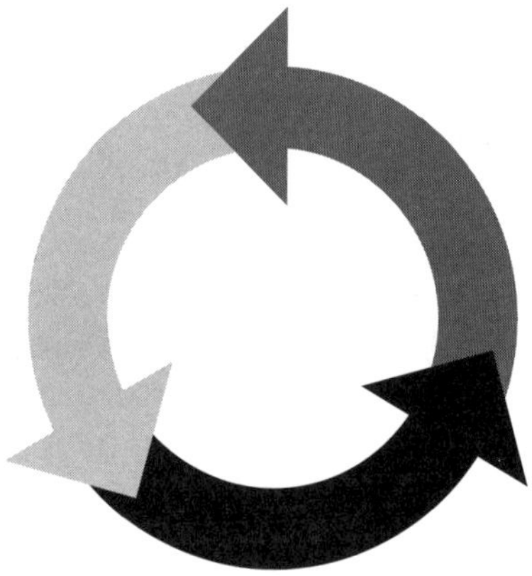

The GIF format also recognizes different types of color palettes. The standard system palette is designed to have a broad range of colors available for the display of whatever image is required. This range is wasted, however, if an image does not have a wide spectrum of colors. For example, a photograph that is primarily made up of shades of blue does not need to be represented by a palette containing various shades of red or green. The computer can automatically adjust the palette to cover the range of colors actually present in the image, and have a different palette for each image. This is known as an *adaptive palette.*

The JPEG compression scheme works by actually removing the description of certain pixels, but in such a way that it is difficult—if not impossible—for the human eye to detect. When saving a file as a JPEG, the user is given a choice of image quality. By turning the image quality down to some degree, smaller files will be obtained, increasing the speed of downloading without giving up much in perceived detail when the image is viewed online.

There is rarely any point in having a graphic on a Web site that will not fit in a browser window and must be scrolled. By keeping your graphics limited to an appropriately small physical size, pixel density, and overall number of images, you will keep your Web pages loading rapidly and make your site quick and responsive. All of these image formats can be manipulated so as to reduce file size further. There are a number of good references on this topic.[4-6]

Animation and Sound

As bandwidth steadily increases, more and more new features are appearing on the Web. It is now possible to provide reasonably high-quality music, animated motion, and even video over the Internet in real time, even to those people with relatively slow dial-up connections to the Internet. These features certainly are a natural enhancement to sites devoted to the music industry, entertainment, or news. Medical sites can also benefit from this technology, which can aid in the education of patients and physicians alike.

Animations can be effective ways of describing complex biological systems or new procedures. Web-based video, audio, or multimedia presentations can provide continuing medical education for physicians as well as public health education for patients. Such presentations can be live, with the opportunity to send questions to the presenter through the Internet, or archived, to allow for study at the convenience of the user. For the most part, however, such features require the services of a Web design professional and the cooperation of the administrator of the computer that hosts the site.

Interactivity

The ability to contact someone through a Web site dramatically increases its utility and appeal, especially in the field of medicine. While any site can be made "interactive" by simply posting an e-mail address, a truly interactive site will enable the user to send messages directly from a Web page, or even engage in real-time, text-based conversation (also known as *chat*) with the site operators.[7] This is a significant advantage, especially for people not fully comfortable with e-mail. In addition, Web-based messaging is easier to make secure than is conventional person-to-person e-mail. Furthermore, some potential patients may be accessing the site through computers where sending e-mail is not easy or even possible—a friend's computer, a public library workstation, a waiting room, or even a freestanding information kiosk. As the Internet becomes more and more a mainstream part of our culture, Web access is becoming ubiquitous. I recently had the opportunity to surf the Web while exercising in a hotel health club, through a touch screen attached to the front of a Stairmaster![8]

The problem with including interactive elements on your practice Web site is that it represents an ongoing commitment of time on the part of whomever is designated to respond. A static site can be a useful addition to a medical practice—once implemented, the only continuing obligation is to make sure that it is appropriately updated whenever something changes in the group (eg, a new physician or new health plan participation). Unanswered e-mail, however, is considered impolite, and may imply a lack of concern on the part of the practice. In today's online world it is better not to have an avenue of communications than to have one that goes unattended. While there are a number of issues that should be addressed before making the site interactive (see Chapter 10), once the channel is opened, responses should be consistent and timely.

Endnotes

1. Flanders V, Willis M. *Web Pages That Suck: Learn Good Design by Looking at Bad Design.* San Francisco, Calif: Sybex; 1998.
2. Kiel JM, Campbell RJ. Designing yourpractice.com: ten steps to an informative website. *MD Comput.* 1999;16:30-33.
3. Dekker F, St John D. *HTML for Beginners.* CNET Web site. Available at: www.builder.com/Authoring/Basics.
4. Litt J. *Web Graphics 101, Part I: Graphic Formats for the Web: GIF, JPG, & PNG.* About Web site. Available at: http://graphicdesign.about.com/arts/graphicdesign/library/weekly/aa012998i.htm.
5. Roelofs G. *PNG: The Definitive Guide.* Sebastopol, Calif: O'Reilly; 1999.
6. Webster T, Atzberger P, Zolli A. *Web Designer's Guide to PNG, GIF, JPEG.* Indianapolis, Ind: Hayden Books; 1997.
7. HumanClick Web site. Available at: www.humanclick.com.
8. Netpulse Web site. Available at: www.netpulse.net/home.html.

Chapter 8
Cohesive Site Creation: Internal and External Linkage

"New links must be forged as old ones rust."

Jane Howard

Linkage between resources is a defining feature of the World Wide Web. Indeed, the Web metaphor itself implies a network of information built from an endless series of links between pages on a site (internal) and between the sites themselves (external). Linking is what makes the Web hypertext (actually, hypermedia) as mentioned previously in Chapter 3. Without linking, the Web is just a very large library. It is therefore important to be extremely careful in constructing links, as errors here can significantly damage the perceived quality of the Web site, frustrate the site visitor, and possibly expose you to legal and ethical problems.

Internal Linkage

The internal structure of a Web site should be one of the first topics considered when constructing an online presence. Even before choices are made regarding the look and feel, time should be taken to visualize the overall flow of information and navigation across the Web site. Just as a house is built from the foundation up, with the framing being done before interior decorating can be considered, the organization of the Web site must be completely mapped out in the initial stages of design.

It should be readily apparent from the home page how to reach every other resource on the Web site. Nothing ensures failure of the site quite like forcing the viewer to hunt for links or use elaborate searching tools to find commonly requested features. It is true that a search feature may be a helpful addition to a content-rich site, especially if the viewer is looking for an obscure piece of information. However, this is no substitute for careful layout and commonsense organization of the key site topics.

Novice Web authors frequently use a flat architecture for their resources, keeping all Web pages and images in one large folder. A better approach is to have a hierarchical file system to organize these elements. This makes it easier to add new sections at a later date, or to make global corrections in a number of files. As long as the internal linkage directions are accurate, the site will appear as intended.

Linking is accomplished by specifying the address of the *link target*—the unique point on the Internet to which the viewer is taken. This can be through absolute or relative references. An *absolute* reference gives the target in terms of its URL (uniform resource locator). For a Web page, the URL will start with the prefix "http://" followed by an identifying string of text that specifies the particular host computer, followed by the location of the target on that computer. A *relative* reference simply gives the name of the page or other file—this presumes that the target is in the same folder on the same computer as the current page. If the target is not in exactly the same folder, but in a subfolder, the name of the subfolder is given first (Figure 8.1).

Figure 8.1

The difference between absolute and relative naming schemes. Web page A is to include a link to the target image B. When using absolute naming, the location of the image is specified by its unique Internet address (URL). Using relative naming, the location of the target image is specified in terms of its relationship to the original Web page.

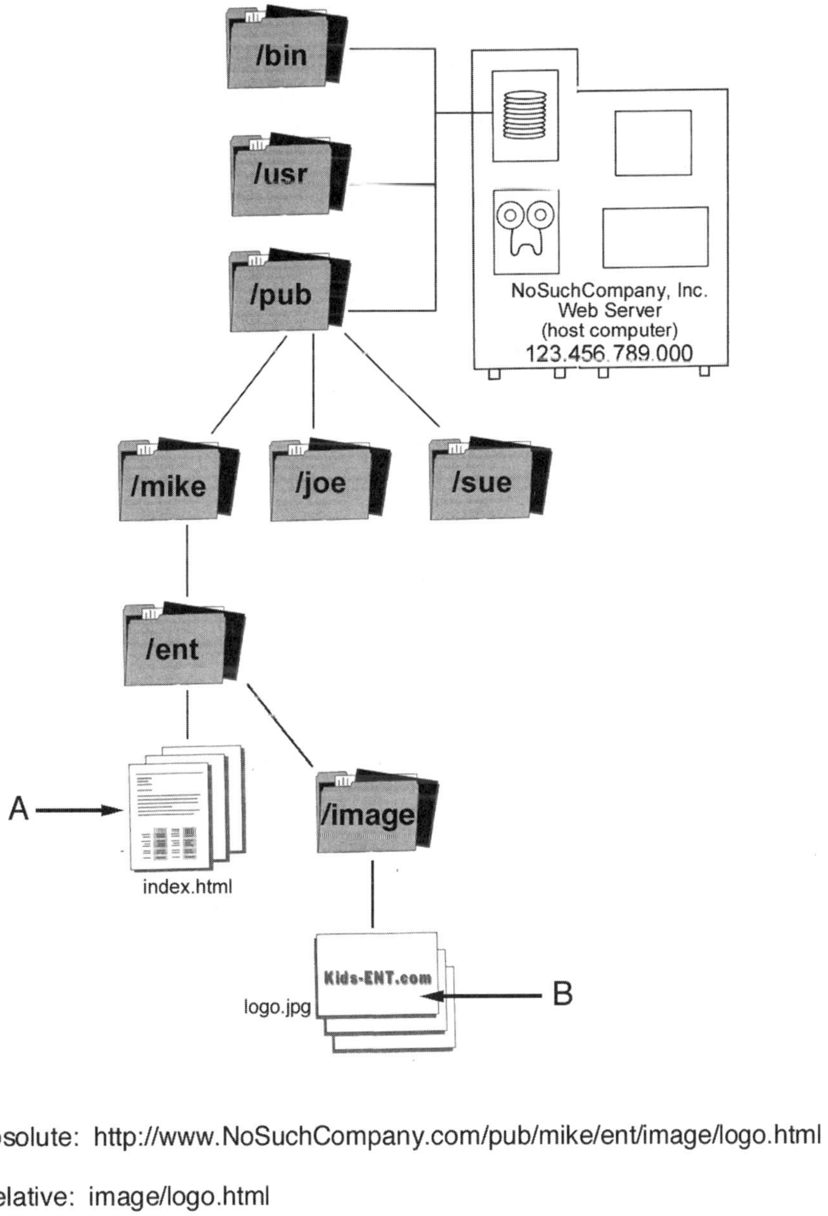

Absolute references clearly must be used for targets outside the current Web site, on other computers (external links). Relative references are preferred for internal links. Although absolute internal links will work initially, if the site is ever moved to another host computer (or to another folder or directory on the original computer), all of the absolute links need to be changed to reflect this move. Relative links do not have this problem, as they only specify position relative to the current page, which will be moved along with all of the other files on the site.

Obviously, it is important that all internal links be carefully checked before launching a site. Having links to nowhere ("dead links") is very poor form, implying a lack of maintenance. It is also confusing for anyone navigating the site. Make sure that all internal links are updated when any organizational rearrangement of the file structure on the site is done, as this can easily produce a large number of dead links. Furthermore, a simple navigation strip at the bottom of the page (Figure 8.2) is helpful, enabling the viewer to quickly move around the site without searching for navigation buttons or continually backing up to previous pages.

Figure 8.2

Navigation links at the bottom of every page on the site. These small items ensure that the viewer can easily escape to any other desired point from any page on the site.

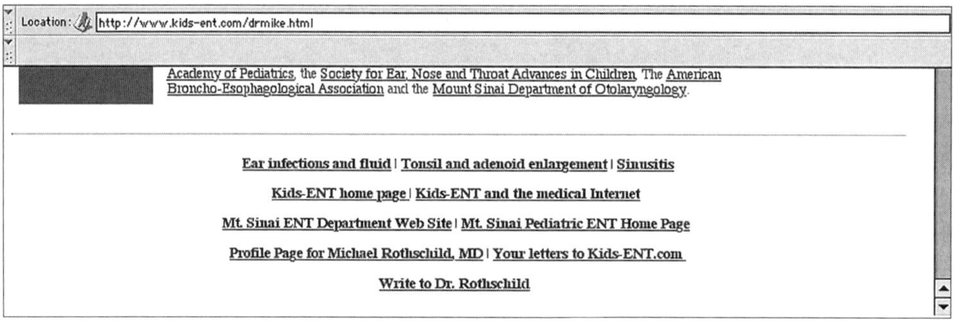

External Linkage

Errors in internal linkage may result in sites that are confusing to navigate or that appear to be unfinished or unprofessional. However, errors in external linkage can have serious legal and ethical repercussions. Linking between globally distributed resources is one of the keys to the Web's utility. Nevertheless, extreme care must be taken when adding links to external Web sites, as an external link is in many ways a tacit endorsement of someone else's content.

A familiar example of a hypertext link is a reference citation in a published article. An author who wishes to cite another work can examine the material, determine whether it is of good quality, appropriate, and relevant, and then refer to it in his or her work. It is certain that the cited reference will always remain as it is, supporting the author's thesis as intended.

A Web site is, however, a dynamic entity. Even if you fully approve of another site and link to it, there is no assurance that it will not change in the future, perhaps in an unwelcome manner. Furthermore, each site to which you link has links of its own. By placing an external link on your page, you are giving an implied endorsement of that site and potentially every site that it endorses in turn. Clearly, care should be taken when constructing such links.

Another concern is the possibility of running afoul of federal laws by linking. Legislation exists to combat "kickback" schemes in which physicians refer to other organizations or businesses in which they have a financial interest.[1] If a medical group has a link to the Web site of a facility to which they refer patients, it is conceivable that health care fraud could be alleged. Alternatively, a hospital that links to the site of a referring physician could be considered to be providing advertising services without charge to one of its "customers."

Another emerging point of concern is the practice of *deep linking*, in which reference is made to a page within another organization's site without passing through the home page or other revenue-generating structure. While this may seem innocuous enough, when high-profile sites are involved, disputes may ensue. Such disputes have erupted into litigation over the past few years, involving Ticketmaster and Microsoft's Seattle Sidewalk, for example, as well as eBay and a number of other auction sites. It is certainly possible for a similar problem to occur in the health arena, especially as medical portals become more prominent and more protective of their content.

Endnote

1. Chin T. Look before you link. *American Medical News*. 2000:30-31.

Chapter 9
Content Development

"The Internet is so big, so powerful and pointless that for some people it is a complete substitute for life."

Andrew Brown, British journalist

Content—the intellectual substance and meaning of any Web site—is the main currency of the online world. Purveyors of Web-based resources are constantly searching for high-quality, current content, and issues of copyright have become prominent as the law moves to deal with intellectual property in this new, easily duplicated form. Furthermore, the daily requirement for Internet content to keep the vast rivers of data filled continues to grow. In this setting, authors have become "content providers," traffickers in a commodity, much as physicians have become "health care providers" to the corporate world of managed care.

There is an Internet aphorism: "Content is king." This was certainly true in the early days of the Web, when images were rudimentary at best, and layout was something of an afterthought. In the current online environment, the balance has shifted. While content still is the key to a valuable medical Web site, form has come to carry more weight. Indeed, certain advertising sites for products or services can succeed merely by setting a mood or raising product awareness with limited content.

Sources of Medical Content

There are two ways of obtaining content for your online presence. You can create it yourself or obtain it elsewhere (either by copying it or through external linking). These are complementary approaches, and each may have a place on a medical practice Web site. Personal practice preferences are best represented in your own words, as you do with postoperative instructions. Furthermore, if you have a unique approach to a disease or a procedure, your own discussion will be a valuable addition to the site. On the other hand, conditions that are handled in a fairly straightforward manner according to established protocols might be better served by using standard discussions or policy statements published by a national medical organization. Most medical societies produce and retain copyright on a significant library of relevant content, and will have a scheme for licensing this material to their members.

It is extremely important that content you create yourself be carefully checked for factual, stylistic, and typographical errors. Unlike peer-reviewed journal articles, where there is some editorial oversight and professional proofreading, you alone are responsible for your online statements. This is clearly not something that can be delegated to your Webmaster or marketing consultant. Before "going live" with any material, it is best to have it read by colleagues within your field for a content assessment, as well as by a number of lay readers to ensure that your writing is understandable to someone who is not a medical professional. Even minor flaws like spelling errors make the site seem unprofessional and can make the content itself suspect.

There are two types of content obtained from secondary sources: static and dynamic. *Static* content would be an article, policy statement, or patient education brochure. While it is certainly possible that this material could change at some point, the expectation is that these types of documents are finished products. Obviously, medicine is constantly changing, and the timeliness and utility of these resources must be reassessed at intervals. If the material is attached to your site by links, periodic alterations might be done by the sponsoring organization. If, on the other hand, you have copied the text (with the appropriate permission and citation) and included it on your own site, it is up to you to make sure that it remains current and accurate.

An example of *dynamic* content is an online news service. Several medical organizations publish breaking stories on a regular basis and provide them to their members through the Web. In this fashion, these medical "wire services" automatically update the content on the member's Web site. Examples of static and dynamic content provided by Medem through a practice Web site are shown in Figure 9.1.

Figure 9.1

Static (A) and dynamic (B) patient information produced by two national medical organizations (the American Medical Association and the American Academy of Pediatrics). This content was made available for use on a physicians' Web site produced through Medem, a company whose sponsoring societies have arranged to share intellectual property with their members in this manner.

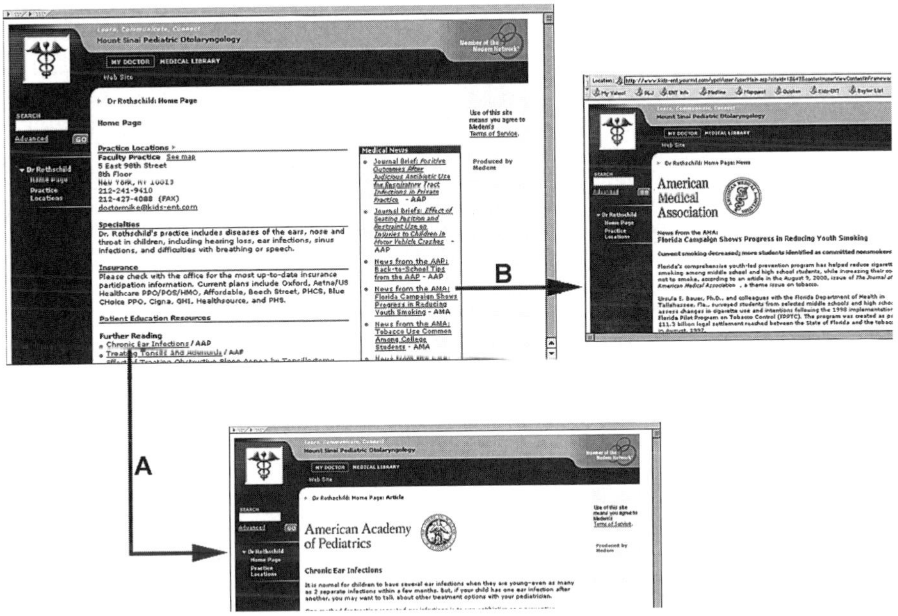

Quality of Content

There is a major ethical issue related to the online dissemination of medical information. From the patient's point of view, it can be difficult to determine whether a discussion of a particular disease or treatment is scientifically sound, up to date, comprehensive, or free from any conflict of interest. In medical literature, we rely on the stature of journals and their editorial staff to act as a quality filter or stamp of approval. There is no analogous institution to "authenticate" medical information distributed online, where anyone can publish anything with ease. Furthermore, there is no legal precedent to support external regulation, and no practical way to accomplish this in any case (given the First Amendment issues and the ease of serving data from overseas computers).

The two best defenses that we can offer against poor-quality medical information of suspect origin are patient education and the adoption of voluntary standards. When discussing health matters, it is important to help patients understand the scientific method and the "red flags" that might indicate suspect information. Patients should understand that it will never be possible for any regulatory body to guarantee the quality of online material, just as medical journal editorial boards cannot guarantee the veracity of their published research. In the same way that we teach medical students and residents to critically evaluate whatever they read—regardless of the source—patients should be helped to understand that the onus is on them to be educated consumers of information. A number of Web-based tools have been developed with this goal in mind.[1,2]

It is important not to be hostile or defensive when patients bring information gleaned from the Internet to the consultation room. Generally, this is a sign of a patient with a desire for knowledge and understanding of his or her condition. Contrary to their reputation of being "difficult patients," most health Web users are more than happy to have their physicians assist them in their online searches. If the material that they have found is suspect, take the opportunity to educate them about criteria for quality Web sites, and be prepared to offer your own recommendations for online information in your specialty.[3]

Voluntary Standards

Several organizations have attempted to compile voluntary standards for medical information on the Internet—these standards are not universal but are certainly a step in the right direction.[4] The Health on the Net Foundation (based in Switzerland) was one of the first of such efforts, releasing the HON code of conduct in 1996.[5] At this point, HON has developed a certification seal, as well as a procedure for site evaluation and the reporting of sites that display the seal but do not seem to conform to the HON standards.

HON Code of Conduct, Health on the Net Foundation, Geneva, Switzerland (The full text can be found at www.hon.ch/HONcode/)

1. ***Authority***
   Any medical or health advice provided and hosted on this site will only be given by medically trained and qualified professionals unless a clear statement is made that a piece of advice offered is from a non-medically qualified individual or organization.

2. ***Complementarity***
   The information provided on this site is designed to support, not replace, the relationship that exists between a patient/site visitor and his/her existing physician.

3. ***Confidentiality***
   Confidentiality of data relating to individual patients and visitors to a medical/health Web site, including their identity, is respected by this Web site. The Web site owners undertake to honor or exceed the legal requirements of medical/health information privacy that apply in the country and state where the Web site and mirror sites are located.

4. ***Attribution***
   Where appropriate, information contained on this site will be supported by clear references to source data and, where possible, have specific HTML links to that data. The date when a clinical page was last modified will be clearly displayed (eg, at the bottom of the page).

5. ***Justifiability***
   Any claims relating to the benefits/performance of a specific treatment, commercial product or service will be supported by appropriate, balanced evidence in the manner outlined above in Principle 4.

6. ***Transparency of authorship***
   The designers of this Web site will seek to provide information in the clearest possible manner and provide contact addresses for visitors that seek further information or support. The Webmaster will display his/her e-mail address clearly throughout the Web site.

7. ***Transparency of sponsorship***
   Support for this Web site will be clearly identified, including the identities of commercial and non-commercial organizations that have contributed funding, services or material for the site.

8. ***Honesty in advertising & editorial policy***
   If advertising is a source of funding it will be clearly stated. A brief description of the advertising policy adopted by the Web site owners will be displayed on the site. Advertising and other promotional material will be presented to viewers in a manner and context that facilitates differentiation between it and the original material created by the institution operating the site.

Several organizations based in the United States have released standards for online health content in 2000, but have yet to produce a certification seal. Hi-Ethics (Health Internet Ethics) is the product of a group of 20 commercial Web ventures, including well-known health-oriented portals such as Medscape and Healtheon/WebMD, in addition to major entities such as America Online and Discovery.com.[6] Hi-Ethics has also announced an agreement with TRUSTe, a nonprofit privacy program that provides a "seal of approval" for appropriate privacy standards for a variety of online resources. Presumably, a certification seal for health sites will be forthcoming from this venture.

The Internet Healthcare Coalition (IHC) is an affiliation of representatives from a number of academic, industry, and advocacy groups.[7] The IHC is oriented toward education of providers and consumers of online health care information, as well as self-regulation of content assisted by the guidelines it is establishing as the eHealth

Code of Ethics. In October of 2000, the three organizations mentioned here (HON, IHC, and Hi-Ethics) announced a collaborative effort to create standards for ethical conduct codes relating to the medical Internet.[8]

Summary of the International e-Health Code of Ethics, Internet Health Care Coalition, May 2000 (Full text available at http://www.ihealthcoalition.org/ethics/ehcode.html)

CANDOR: Disclose information that if known by consumers would likely affect consumers' understanding or use of the site or purchase or use of a product or service (eg, financial relationships, conflicts of interest, site purpose).

HONESTY: Be truthful and not deceptive. Information should be presented in a forthright manner without being misleading.

QUALITY: Provide health information that is accurate, easy to understand and up to date. A good faith effort should be made to evaluate, maintain and fully explain the information presented. True medical controversy should be acknowledged, and information should be labeled as the result of scientific studies, expert consensus or personal opinion. Users should be provided with information needed to draw their own conclusions about the content of the site.

INFORMED CONSENT: Respect the users' right to determine whether or how their personal data may be collected, used or shared.

PRIVACY: Respect the obligation to protect users' privacy. Reasonable steps should be taken to prevent unauthorized access to or use of personal data.

PROFESSIONALISM: Respect fundamental ethical obligations to patients and clients, as established by medical tradition and all applicable laws concerning health care. Inform and educate patients and clients about the limitations of online health care.

RESPONSIBLE PARTNERING: Ensure that any affiliated organizations and sites are trustworthy.

ACCOUNTABILITY: Provide meaningful opportunity for users to give feedback to the site, and monitor compliance with the eHealth Code of Ethics.

The AMA has also compiled an extensive policy statement that was published in the *Journal of the American Medical Association* and is available online.[9,10] This document is intended to apply to AMA Internet publications. However, it is a good example of a thorough and specific policy for academic medical online publishing in general, and goes into considerably more depth than other guidelines mentioned previously.

Trust is perhaps the most valuable commodity on the medical Internet. Patients do recognize that all content is not the same, and are looking for guidance in their searching. Interestingly (and reassuringly), people seem to trust information obtained from their own doctors more than that obtained from a large health care portal or medical organization. This is supported by research that demonstrates the importance of prior face-to-face contact when establishing successful online relationships,[11] and by study reports that almost three quarters of those seeking online health information would trust sites recommended by their doctors.[12]

Content is the heart of any online presence. It is the value that you can provide to your established and potential patients that will keep them coming back to your pages. By adhering to the highest ethical standards and continually ensuring and maintaining the quality of your content, you will provide an appreciated service to your site visitors. The trust that you establish in person can carry over to your Web site, and high-quality information online will enhance your professional image and your relationships with your patients.

Endnotes

1. Discern questionnaire. Discern Web site. Available at: www.discern.org.uk.
2. Quality Information Checklist. Quick Web site. Available at: www.quick.org.uk.
3. Chin T. Site reading: Physicians grapple with recommending Web sites. *American Medical News*. October 23/30, 2000:22-23.
4. Foubister V. Web rules. *American Medical News*. July 31, 2000:11-12.
5. Health on the Net Foundation Web site. Available at: www.hon.ch.
6. Hi-Ethics. Health Internet Ethics Web site. Available at: www.hiethics.com.
7. Internet Healthcare Coalition Web site. Available at: www.ihc.net.
8. Top e-Health Ethics Groups Announce Collaboration. Internet Healthcare Coalition Web site. Available at: www.ihealthcoalition.org/about/ihc_pr9.html.
9. Winker MA, Flanagin A, Chi-Lum B, et al. Guidelines for medical and health information sites on the internet: principles governing AMA web sites. *JAMA*. 2000;283:1600-1606.
10. Principles governing AMA publications web sites. American Medical Association Web site. Available at: http://pubs.ama-assn.org/ama_web.html.
11. Slade M. On the global, faceless web, trust counts for even more. *New York Times*. March 29, 2000.
12. CyberCitizen Health 2000. Cyber Dialog Web site. Available at: www.cyberdialogue.com/resource/press/releases/2000/08-22-cch-launch.html.

Chapter 10

Online Doctor-Patient Relationships and Cybermedicine

"Electric communication will never be a substitute for the face of someone who with their soul encourages another person to be brave and true."

Charles Dickens

Up to this point, we have focused on the one-way dissemination of information from doctor to patient using the Internet. However, any physician with an Internet presence must decide whether or not to participate in online dialogue, either with established patients, or with Web site visitors who have never been seen in person. This question generates considerable anxiety and controversy with regard to medical practice Web sites. In many ways, e-mail and other types of online correspondence are similar to prior modes of doctor-patient communication. However, there are also many unique aspects of this channel that require rethinking the classic legal and ethical context of, for example, the telephone.[1] There are a number of approaches to online communication between doctor and patient, ranging from the most conservative (refusing such contact) to the most open and inclusive.

Limited Online Communication

Simply by not posting an e-mail address or by not having a Web-based message submission feature on the Web site, a doctor can preclude any online contact by site visitors. Some may feel that this is a noticeable absence, and worry that the lack of an e-mail address will seem inappropriately distant. However, if the site itself provides valuable content, there is no reason to feel pressured to encourage online communication. Site visitors certainly have the option of conventional telephone contact should they wish to establish a doctor-patient relationship.

Another option would be to only enable contact with the Webmaster, intended for the submission of comments or complaints about the site itself, and not about medical issues. This is an acceptable approach; however, some protocol should be established for the inevitable clinical question or request. Such queries could be answered with a standard response, making a referral to the appropriate offline contact person.

Online Communication With Established Patients

Some physicians allow online communication between established patients and the office, but refuse such contact with individuals not known to the practice. This can be achieved by giving patients who visit the office a password-protected account, or an e-mail address that does not appear on the Web site. Such an approach may be particularly appealing, because the patients realize that they are being given special access to the office staff. If this communication is done through a Web site (as opposed to standard e-mail), a greater degree of privacy can be assured. Web sites can be made fairly secure, and do not require the use of any special e-mail encryption software by the patient, which is difficult to employ with an ever-expanding patient population using a variety of computers and Internet connections.

While certainly there are concerns and controversies about its proper use,[1-4] online communication is a good substitute for "phone tag" about nonurgent matters, in which both the doctor and the patient can correspond at a convenient time. Furthermore, it is self-documenting, as the messages can be printed out and included in the paper chart. Communication of a more "clerical" nature has been successfully integrated into medical practices through Web sites or e-mail schemes, facilitating tasks such as appointment scheduling, requests for prescription refills, or billing inquiries. The legal status of this type of messaging is in many ways similar to that of a telephone call. Unlike telephone communications, however, both parties (the doctor and the patient) potentially have a physical and/or electronic document that records the exact date, time, and content of the exchange. While it is a legal requirement (and good practice) to document all phone calls in the medical chart, it is much less likely that telephone conversations will be recorded in a complete and unbiased manner by either person.

It is crucial that security and privacy issues are explicitly addressed when corresponding with patients electronically (see Figure 10.1). Some physicians have even developed formal printed consent forms to be signed before engaging in this type of online communication. Patients need to know that confidential information may be contained in your replies. Family members who share a single e-mail account are at risk for a significant breach of privacy. Patients must also understand how e-mail or Web-based communication is handled in the office, who has access to these messages, when a reply will be sent, and when to use the telephone (eg, emergencies).[5,6] There is legal precedent for malpractice based on the failure to return a telephone call in a timely manner.[7] It is clearly good practice to firmly establish the expected turnaround time for e-mail before encouraging your patients to use this technology.

Figure 10.1

A sample e-mail exchange. Note the disclaimer included in the text of the reply as well as at the end of the message.

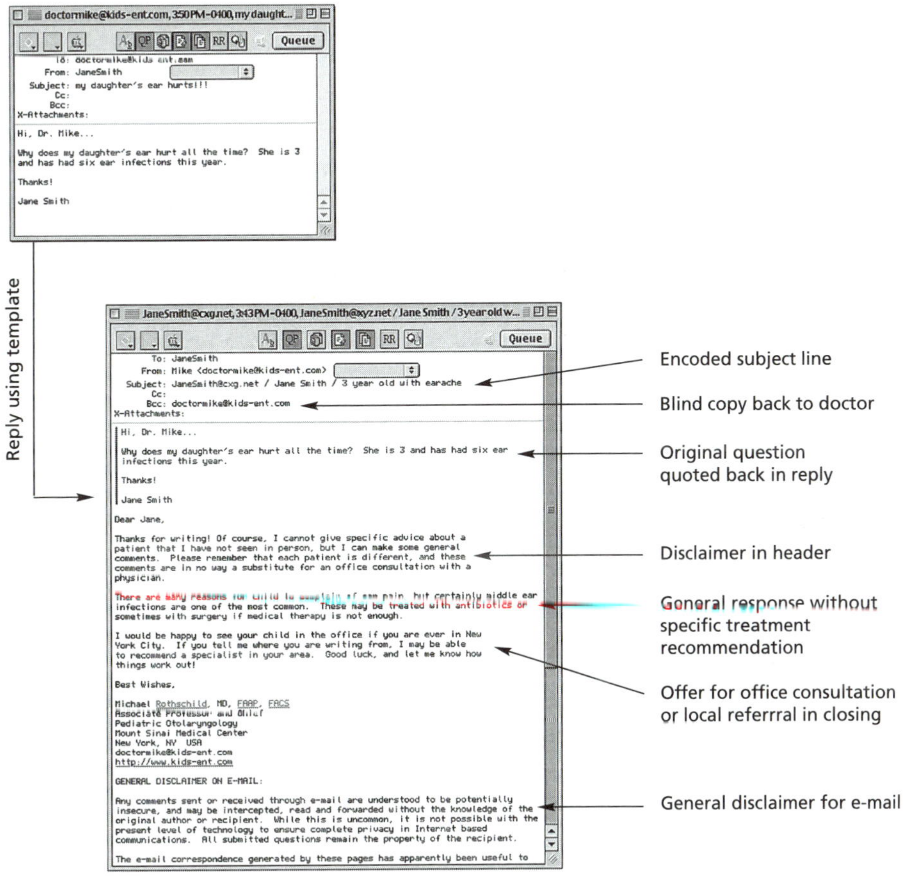

AMA Guidelines for Patient-Physician Electronic Mail[6]

H-478.997 Guidelines for Patient-Physician Electronic Mail

(1) For those physicians who choose to utilize e-mail for selected patient and medical practice communications, the following guidelines be adopted.

Communication Guidelines: (a) Establish turnaround time for messages. Exercise caution when using e-mail for urgent matters. (b) Inform patient about privacy issues. Patients should know: (c) Who besides addressee processes messages during addressee's usual business hours and during addressee's vacation or illness; and (d) That the message may be included as part of the medical record, at the discretion of the physician. (e) Establish types of transactions (prescription refill, appointment scheduling, etc.) and sensitivity of subject matter (HIV, mental health, etc.) permitted over e-mail. (f) Instruct patients to put the category of transaction in the subject line of the message for filtering: prescription, appointment, medical advice, billing question. (g) Request that patients put their name and patient identification number in the body of the message. (h) Configure automatic reply to acknowledge receipt of messages. (i) Print all messages, with replies and confirmation of receipt, and place in patient's paper chart. (j) Send a new message to inform patient of completion of request. (k) Request that patients use autoreply feature to acknowledge reading clinician's message. (l) Develop archival and retrieval mechanisms. (m) Maintain a mailing list of patients, but do not send group mailings where recipients are visible to each other. Use blind copy feature in software. (n) Avoid anger, sarcasm, harsh criticism, and libelous references to third parties in messages.

Medicolegal and Administrative Guidelines: (a) Develop a patient-clinician agreement for the informed consent for the use of e-mail. This should be discussed with the patient and documented in the medical record. Agreement should contain the following: (b) Terms in communication guidelines (stated above). (c) Provide instructions for when and how to convert to phone calls and office visits. (d) Describe security mechanisms in place. (e) Hold harmless the health care institution for information loss due to technical failures. (f) Waive encryption requirement, if any, at patient's insistence. (g) Describe security mechanisms in place including: (h) Using a password-protected screen saver for all desktop workstations in the office, hospital, and at home. (i) Never forwarding patient-identifiable information to a third party without the patient's express permission. (j) Never using patient's e-mail address in a marketing scheme. (k) Not sharing professional e-mail accounts with family members. (l) Not using unencrypted wireless communications with patient-identifiable information. (m) Double-checking all "To" fields prior to sending messages. (n) Perform at least weekly backups of e-mail onto long-term storage. Define long-term as the term applicable to paper records. (o) Commit policy decisions to writing and electronic form.

(2) The policies and procedures for e-mail be communicated to all patients who desire to communicate electronically.

(3) The policies and procedures for e-mail be applied to facsimile communications, where appropriate. (BOT Rep. 2, A-00)

Standard Disclaimer Attached to the End of the Author's E-Mail Responses to Established Patients

GENERAL DISCLAIMER ON E-MAIL

Established patients (and parents of patients) from Dr. Rothschild's practice should feel free to use e-mail for non-urgent matters (the mail is checked fairly frequently). However, If there is an emergency, please use the office number (212 241-9410), which is answered 24 hours a day, seven days a week.

It must be understood that any comments sent or received through e-mail are potentially insecure, and may be intercepted, read and forwarded without the knowledge of the original author or recipient. While this is uncommon, it is not possible with the present level of technology to ensure complete privacy in Internet based communications.

Cybermedicine and Teleadvice

The most open approach to online doctor-patient communication is to provide the opportunity for the general Internet community to submit medical questions and receive personalized answers. Such unsolicited requests (or "cold questions") are common once an online presence is made public. Questions can be submitted by e-mail, or through the Web site itself using a comment submission form. Certainly, this is of considerable value to site visitors. I have answered many such e-mail inquiries through the Kids-ENT.com site, and have always been impressed by the earnest and forthright nature of the requests, as well as the gratitude expressed by a large number of correspondents.

Providing personalized comments in a timely fashion without charge is a sure way to make your Web site extremely popular. It is tempting to answer simple questions and "make the diagnosis"—perhaps this is a vestigial response left over from our days of medical student roundsmanship! One study found that of 58 physicians maintaining Web sites, 50% responded to a fictitious inquiry, with only nine of these refusing to make any advice without seeing the patient in person.[8] This is one way to market a medical practice; answering such questions may well bring new patients into the office. I have had a number of patients come in for a consultation after I had answered their unsolicited e-mail, including several from distant states and even from overseas.

Despite the presumed benefits to the practice (good will and marketing) and the obvious benefits to those who write for advice, there are many concerns about the risks of answering such requests. Most of these concerns center on the potential liability for bad outcomes or for practicing medicine in a state or country where the physician is not licensed. The central question in this new type of interchange is what exactly constitutes a doctor-patient relationship, with its attendant responsibilities.

The term "telemedicine" simply means the use of any sort of telecommunications device to diagnose and treat a patient.[9] The newer term "cybermedicine" has a somewhat different connotation, referring to the open exchange of ideas online without necessarily involving doctor-patient relationships. Cybermedicine is based more on promoting education and public health, as opposed to specific interventions on the behalf of individual patients.[10] It is a broader field than telemedicine, including aspects of marketing, casual advice, communication between patients, the sale of drugs or devices, and the creation of new relationships.[11]

There is certainly nothing new about telemedicine—in fact, in the 17th and 18th centuries, the preferred method of diagnosis was through written descriptions of symptoms received by mail or other messenger. It was not until the middle of the 19th century that the physical examination was seen as a necessary part of the doctor-patient relationship.[7] The telegraph, and subsequently the telephone, have since been utilized to provide for consultation without the inconvenience of a physical visit, but most doctors recognize the limitations of such remote interactions with their patients. A major fear has been the exposure to claims of medical malpractice related to health care delivered without the full benefit of an office or bedside encounter.

Clearly, every doctor who has phoned in a prescription or told a caller to come to the office in the morning has engaged in a type of telemedicine. It is simply not practical for most doctors to completely avoid this activity. As the Internet radically changes and greatly enhances our communications abilities, these questions will become more and more prominent. Therefore, it is worthwhile to consider the actual risks involved in all types of doctor-patient communication, and make an informed choice as to your degree of participation.

Legal Concerns

Traditionally, medical malpractice involves three features: the existence of a duty to care for a patient, the breach of this duty by not meeting established standards of care, and the presence of demonstrable damages.[9] The first of these is the one that has generated the most controversy in the medical Internet. A duty to care can only exist if there is an established doctor-patient relationship. Therefore, if litigation occurs, the courts may determine on an individual basis whether or not a doctor-patient relationship existed.

Such a determination is usually based on the degree to which the physician applied his or her judgment to the patient's case, and whether the patient accepted that judgment as applicable to his or her particular situation. Casual conversation in a social setting is not necessarily considered the grounds for a doctor-patient relationship. The mere fact that a patient had contact with a physician and described symptoms (eg, through the telephone) does not necessarily imply that such a relationship is formed. The test must be whether the doctor agreed to professionally advise the patient and whether the patient relied on this advice in some way. For the patient to have relied on the advice, it must have been the basis for action (or inaction, in the case of reassurance).[9] Clearly, if a doctor gives specific advice, a diagnosis, or recommendations for management, a doctor-patient relationship may have been established whether or not a fee is charged or a face-to-face consultation has occurred.[1,12] On the other hand, a doctor providing general medical content on a Web site no more establishes a doctor-patient relationship with his audience than does the author of a published article or a speaker at a public conference.[11,13]

It is not clear at present what the legal and ethical status is of intermediate-type cybermedicine relationships, in which general explanations of a disease state or a physician referral is given in response to a request for information. This type of communication has been termed "teleadvice," as opposed to "telemedicine"—the latter implying the establishment or furthering of a doctor-patient relationship without physical contact. Most guidelines for telemedicine stress the importance of prior personal contact and the limitations of management from afar. On the other hand, there are few published guidelines covering teleadvice, no specific legislation, and little applicable case law. As of this writing, I am not aware of any successful litigation involving malpractice based solely on e-mail or other Internet communications. Furthermore, the legal system and the legislatures are struggling to apply established case law and statute to these new areas, as well as carefully crafting new opinions and legislation to deal with the unique aspects of cybermedicine.[11]

One of the most ambitious and exhaustive projects to date in this field is the set of guidelines recently released by the eRisk Working Group for Healthcare. This group is a self-regulation effort by a consortium of interested parties, including the previously mentioned Medem Corporation,[12] national medical societies, and 30 medical malpractice carriers (which insure over 70% of the covered physicians in the United States). The outline of these guidelines is presented later in this chapter, while the full document is available online.[14] This recommendation is fairly dense reading, based on an educated analysis of existing law. It should be remembered, however, that evolving legislation, government policy, and judicial decisions will continue to shape the legal status of online doctor-patient communication in the years to come.

Outline of Detailed Guidelines for Managing Risks Associated With Physician-Patient Online Interaction

VERSION 1.0, November 1, 2000, released January 8, 2001

A Work Product of the eRisk in Healthcare Project of the eRisk Working Group for Healthcare.

Contact info: eRisk Working Group for Healthcare, c/o Medem, Inc., 333 Bush, 24th Floor, San Francisco, CA 94104; eRisk@medem.com

1 Introduction

2 Policy and Procedure Guidelines for Provider Organizations

2.1 General Guidelines
2.2 Information Referrals
2.3 Publication of Web Sites
2.4 Use of Shared Provider-Patient Databases
2.5 Use of Online Compliance Tools
2.6 Use of Messaging Services
2.7 Use of Online Communities

3 Guidelines for Individual Provider Policies and Procedures

3.1 General Guidelines
3.2 Information Referrals
3.3 Publication of Web Sites
3.4 Use of Shared Provider-Patient Databases
3.5 Use of Online Compliance Tools
3.6 Use of Messaging Services
3.7 Use of Online Communities

4 Guidelines for Vendors of Online Services

4.1 Privacy, Confidentiality, and Information Security
4.2 Clinical Content
4.3 Physician / Provider Organization Web Sites
4.4 Non-Provider Organization Web Sites
4.5 Provider-Patient Shared Database Applications
4.6 Online Patient Compliance / Disease Management Tools
4.7 Provider-Patient Message-Oriented Communications
4.8 Online Communities
4.9 (reserved)
4.10 Other General, Ethical, Legal, and Liability Considerations

5 Guidelines for Healthcare Information Consumers

6 (reserved)

7 Issues Requiring Political Action

8	***Appendices***
8.1	*Sample "Our Policy for Online Interaction" (Patient Instruction)*
8.2	*Sample "Patient Consent to Treatment by Telemedicine" (California)*
8.3	*Sample "Provider Organization Policy for Online Interaction"*
8.4	*Sample "Provider Organization Contingency Plan for Loss of Online Service"*
8.5	*Sample "Online Patient Identity Authentication Policy"*
8.6	*Sample "Electronic Message Medical Disclaimer Notices"*
8.7	*Sample "Individual Provider Staff Online Interaction Policy"*
8.8	*Other Sources of Guidelines and Information*

Most physicians choose not to respond to teleadvice requests in order to limit potential liability and out of a reluctance to spend time answering questions without the possibility of reimbursement. Even though I only need to spend a few minutes answering each question, and have developed boilerplate text for many common inquiries, getting five or six questions a day can take up a significant amount of time. Other physicians have had similar experiences with this unreimbursed service.[15] And while the lack of a consulting fee does not preclude the presence of a doctor-patient relationship, it is certain that any attempt by the doctor to profit financially (through direct billing or perhaps even on-site advertising) raises the likelihood that a court would find that such a relationship existed.

Positive Aspects of Teleadvice

Teleadvice is appealing from the patient's viewpoint. Patients may be frustrated with conventional avenues of health care, be unwilling to accept a poor prognosis, lack trust in their own doctor's clinical skills or communications abilities, or simply wish to remain anonymous and avoid bringing up certain issues with their physician for a variety of reasons.[16] It is increasingly clear that there is a significant market for health care providers who make themselves accessible through the Internet.

Despite the understandable concerns, there is a case to be made for a nonspecific but helpful response to teleadvice requests.[15,17,18] Not every communication between a physician and another person necessarily constitutes a doctor-patient relationship. There is a huge demand for this type of service in the world today, and to ignore it totally may not be the best long-term solution. One model for the appropriate use of teleadvice is the AMA's policy on physician advisory or referral services by telecommunication. Although developed in 1994 for telephone and the broadcast media, these guidelines describe a reasonable compromise between the needs of the patient and those of the physician dispensing advice online.

AMA Policy on Physician Advisory or Referral Services by Telecommunication[19]

E-5.025 Physician Advisory or Referral Services by Telecommunications.

Telecommunication advisory services, by way of phone, fax or computer, distinct from an existing patient-physician relationship can be a helpful source of medical information for the public. Often, people are not sure where to turn for information of a general medical nature or do not have easy access to other sources of information. Individuals also may be embarrassed about directly bringing up certain questions with their physicians. Although telecommunication advisory services can provide only limited medical services, they can be a useful complement to more comprehensive services, if used properly.

Any telecommunication advisory service should employ certain safeguards to prevent misuse. For example, the physician responding to the call should not make a clinical diagnosis. Diagnosis by telecommunication is done without the benefit of a physician examination or even a face-to-face meeting with the caller. Critical medical data may be unavailable to the physician. Physicians who respond to callers should therefore act within the limitations of telecommunication services and ensure that callers understand the limitations of the services. Under no circumstances should medications be prescribed.

Physicians who respond to the calls should elicit all necessary information from the callers. When callers are charged by the minute, they may try to hurry their calls to limit their costs. As a result, important information may not be disclosed to the physician. Physicians should also ensure that callers do not incur large bills inadvertently or without understanding the billing system.

Physician referral services can also offer important information to the public. Referral services are often provided by medical societies, hospitals and for-profit entities. To ensure that the service bases its recommendation on medically legitimate considerations rather than the likelihood of being paid by the physician, when the service charges physicians a fee to participate, physicians should not pay the service per referral. Also, callers should be told how the list is created. For example, callers should be informed whether the list includes physicians who pay a flat fee to be listed, members of a particular hospital staff or medical society, or physicians who meet some general quality-based criteria.

While these safeguards are described as applying primarily to telephone services, they should be considered equally applicable to any other communication media, such as radio or television in which the physician and patient do not meet face-to-face.

(I, IV, VI) Issued June 1994; Updated June 1996.

If you do choose to answer "cold" questions and provide teleadvice, be sure to maintain the highest ethical standards. Avoid specific recommendations or diagnoses. Rather, use general statements about patients with similar conditions and always use an appropriate disclaimer attached to any online communication (see "The Difference Between Telemedicine and Teleadvice" on this page, and "Sample Response Template and Disclaimer for Teleadvice" on page 84). Be careful not to comment on the management or therapeutic decisions made by other practitioners—you will generally not have the entire story, and a negative comment could result in charges of libel! If I feel that someone's health is being truly compromised, I may diplomatically suggest a second opinion and offer to give the correspondent a referral in his or her geographic area. Keep copies of all correspondence. A Web site visitor should have to accept your disclaimers and guidelines for advice (by clicking on an "I agree" button) before being allowed to read specific information, and certainly before being allowed to send in a question. This documents your effort to ensure that the nature of the advice is understood by the recipient. Finally, you may want to provide an avenue for offline contact when appropriate if the patient chooses to see you in person.

The Difference Between Telemedicine and Teleadvice

Note that the qualifying words in the telemedicine response ("probably," "likely") do not preclude the establishment of a doctor-patient relationship:

Question: "Doctor, my daughter has had two ear infections since the summer, and she has had fluid in her ears for the past 4 months. I am worried that she can't hear me, and she has had two tests that show that she is having a problem hearing. Do you think that she should have ear tube surgery?"

Telemedicine Answer: *"Your daughter probably has a condition known as eustachian tube disfunction (ETD). Since her ear fluid has lasted for 4 months and she has hearing loss, she would likely benefit from this operation. You can find out more about the risks and benefits of tube placement on my Web site, but if you want to schedule a visit to talk about it, feel free to call my office."*

Teleadvice Answer: *"Children who have had fluid for more than 3 months, especially if hearing loss is present, are often candidates for tube surgery. This has been published in a number of medical journals, and while still controversial, seems to be a standard and successful way of managing the very common ear disease of childhood. If you like, I can give you the name of a specialist in your area to examine your daughter and see if she would benefit from the operation."*

Sample Response Template and Disclaimer for Teleadvice

Dear <<NAME>>

Thanks for writing! Of course, I cannot give specific advice about a patient whom I have not seen in person, but I can make some general comments. Please remember that each patient is different, and these comments are in no way a substitute for an office consultation with a physician.

<<RESPONSE>>

I would be happy to see your child in the office if you are ever in New York City. If you tell me where you are writing from, I may be able to recommend a specialist in your area. Good luck, and let me know how things work out!

Best Wishes,
Michael Rothschild, MD, FAAP, FACS
Associate Professor and Chief
Pediatric Otolaryngology
Mount Sinai Medical Center
New York, NY USA
doctormike@kids-ent.com
http://www.kids-ent.com

GENERAL DISCLAIMER ON E-MAIL:

While Dr Rothschild is happy to answer general questions about pediatric ear, nose, and throat problems as time allows, it is important that several points be understood. Any comments made about patients who have not been seen by Dr Rothschild in person are provided as general information only, and should not be considered as advice for a specific child. Every patient is different, and requires individualized management by a health care provider who has been able to meet and examine him or her in person. An exchange of e-mail correspondence over the Internet does not constitute a doctor-patient relationship.

The e-mail correspondence generated by these pages has apparently been useful to parents and other caregivers in helping them to better understand their children's health problems, but it is no substitute for personal medical care. It should also be understood that many topics in medicine are controversial, and there may be several appropriate alternative approaches to a given problem.

E-mail correspondents accept full responsibility for the use of information obtained in this manner. No representation is made as to its completeness or appropriateness for a particular purpose. Dr Rothschild is neither responsible nor liable for any claim, loss, or damage resulting from use of information received solely through e-mail, without an in-person consultation. The mention of a specific product or service does not constitute a recommendation unless so stated.

No change should be made in a health care regimen solely on the basis of information obtained over the Internet, but only after consultation with a health care provider who has had the opportunity to evaluate the patient in person.

Any correspondence submitted to Dr Rothschild may occasionally be used elsewhere for the purpose of illustrating commonly asked questions. However, identifying information (such as names or geographic locations) will not be included. Unsolicited correspondence remains the property of Dr Rothschild, and no other copyright may be implied or reserved.

Finally, it must be understood that any comments sent or received through e-mail are potentially insecure, and may be intercepted, read, and forwarded without the knowledge of the original author or recipient. While this is uncommon, it is not possible with the present level of technology to ensure complete privacy in Internet-based communications.

The following is a simple scheme I have developed to archive responses to e-mail. Note that in general, e-mail cannot be made as secure as Web-based messaging, and evolving standards are moving away from e-mail as a standard for online doctor-patient communication.

- Click "respond" to generate outgoing mail with the original message quoted back to the sender.
- Use a template for responses if possible to include your standard opening paragraph, closing paragraph, and disclaimer.
- In the subject line, enter the e-mail address from which the query was sent, the name of the author (if given), and the topic of the e-mail, separated by "/."
- Send a blind copy to yourself.
- When you receive the copy, you will have in one document the question and your response. Store these copies in a secure location with regular backup. You can use the subject line to group together serial messages from the same author, or to search for particular interchanges by name or topic.

The following are points to consider before providing teleadvice in response to unsolicited e-mail from unknown persons:

1. Think carefully before responding at all (you are under no obligation).
2. Include an appropriate disclaimer, both at the end of the message and as a part of the message itself.
3. Keep records of all such communication (some of these correspondents may become office patients).
4. Answer in general terms, avoiding specific diagnoses or treatment recommendations.
5. Avoid making comments about care already delivered.
6. Offer to see the patient in your office, or recommend a physician in the patient's area, if possible.
7. Be courteous and professional in your responses at all times.

Evolving Standards

As discussed in Chapter 4, the Health Insurance Portability and Accountability Act (HIPAA) and other upcoming privacy regulations will have a major impact on many facets of the health care industry. Providers and payers are increasingly moving to electronic claim submission and processing, thus falling under the jurisdiction of these regulations. However, it is not clear at this point to what extent this law will affect online doctor-patient communication. Clearly, it is in the best interest of both physicians and patients to maintain secure and private communication when using e-mail, just as it would be inappropriate for a doctor to leave the results of a biopsy or HIV test on an answering machine. However, online communication frequently occurs through a variety of less than secure channels, and this trend is increasing. Although in general, Web-based communication can be made more secure than standard e-mail, Web browsers at information kiosks, laptop computers, or Internet-enabled cell phones, pagers, and handheld devices are less likely to be universally secure than the established unchanging communications link between, for example, a billing office and an insurance company.

Over the next few years, as security and privacy standards become enforceable law, protocols for online doctor-patient communication will evolve. It is difficult to predict what compromise of security and convenience will emerge from the dialogue between the government, physicians, patient advocacy groups, and other interested parties. At present, there is considerable interest in the use of various public and private key encryption schemes to enhance the privacy of online communications, but these have yet to be standardized.[20,21] Biometrics approaches to the authentication of users have also begun to surface, using fingerprints, retina scans, or other technology to ensure that sensitive medical information is not released to unauthorized individuals, and that an access audit trail is maintained.[22] Despite these advantages, a cautious, commonsense approach should be used whenever communicating with patients.

Endnotes

1. Spielberg AR. On call and online: sociohistorical, legal, and ethical implications of e-mail for the patient-physician relationship [see comments]. *JAMA*. 1998;280:1353-1359.
2. Jackler RK. Brave new world. *Arch Otolaryngol Head Neck Surg*. 1999;125:471-472.
3. Howard ML. E-mail: effective if handled with care [comment]. *Arch Otolaryngol Head Neck Surg*. 1999;125:471.
4. Kuppersmith RB. Is e-mail an effective medium for physician-patient interactions? *Arch Otolaryngol Head Neck Surg*. 1999;125:468-470.
5. Kane B, Sands DZ. Guidelines for the clinical use of electronic mail with patients. The AMIA Internet Working Group, Task Force on Guidelines for the Use of Clinic-Patient Electronic Mail. *J Am Med Inform Assoc*. 1998;5:104-111.

6. Guidelines for Patient-Physician Electronic Mail. American Medical Association Web site. Available at: www.ama-assn.org/apps/pf_online/pf_online?f_n=resultLink&doc=policyfiles/HOD/H-478.997.HTM&s_t=e-mail&catg=AMA/CnB&catg=AMA/CEJA&catg=AMA/HOD&&nth=1&&st_p=0&nth=2&.
7. Spielberg AR. Online without a net: physician-patient communication by electronic mail. *Am J Law Med.* 1999;25:267-295.
8. Eysenbach G, Diepgen TL. Responses to unsolicited patient e-mail requests for medical advice on the world wide web [see comments]. *JAMA.* 1998;280:1333-1335.
9. Kuszler PC. Telemedicine and integrated health care delivery: compounding malpractice liability. *Am J Law Med.* 1999;25:297-326.
10. Eysenbach G, Sa ER, Diepgen TL. The impact of informatics: shopping around the internet today and tomorrow: towards the millennium of cybermedicine. *BMJ.* 1999;319:1294.
11. Terry NP. Cyber-malpractice: legal exposure for cybermedicine. *Am J Law Med.* 1999;25:327-366.
12. Neill R. Doctor, you've got e-mail [letter; comment]. *JAMA.* 1999;282:730 731.
13. De Ville KA. Internet listservers and pediatrics: newly emerging legal and clinical practice issues. II. *Pediatrics.* 1996;98:453-454.
14. eRisk Guidelines for Physician-Patient Online Communications. Medem Web site. Available at: http://www.medem.com/erisk.html
15. Borowitz SM, Wyatt JC. The origin, content, and workload of e-mail consultations [see comments]. *JAMA.* 1998;280:1321-1324.
16. Eysenbach G, Diepgen TL. Patients looking for information on the internet and seeking teleadvice: motivation, expectations, and misconceptions as expressed in e-mails sent to physicians. *Arch Dermatol.* 1999;135:151-156.
17. Lewis AD. Patients, physicians, and e-mail [letter; comment]. *Arch Dermatol.* 2000;136:121-122.
18. Toub D. Answering medical questions online. *Medicine on the Net.* 2000;6:10.
19. E-5.025 Physician Advisory or Referral Services by Telecommunications. American Medical Association Web site. Available at: www.ama-assn.org/apps/pf_online/pf_online?f_n=browse&doc=policyfiles/CEJA/E-5.025.HTM.
20. van Dyk J. Public key infrastructure: securing the exchange of health information. *MD Comput.* 2000;17:44-46
21. Chin T. Electronic signatures: digital scrawl. *American Medical News.* 2000.
22. The Biometric Consortium. The Biometric Consortium Web site. Available at: http://www.biometrics.org.

Chapter 11
Domain Registration and Hosting

"A good name is better than precious ointment."

Ecclesiastes 7:1

The Uniform Resource Locator

All resources available online (such as Web pages) must have a unique identifying "address" so that they can be retrieved from any computer connected to the Internet. This address is known as the *uniform resource locator* (URL). The URL consists of three parts: the resource type, the domain name, and the pathway to the specific resource (see Figure 11.1).

The most common resource type today is "http://", which designates that the resource is a Web page. There are other resource types, but they are rarely seen by most Internet users. The domain name follows the resource type, and specifies the computer on which the resource is stored. A computer that stores a resource and makes it accessible through the Internet is said to be *hosting* the resource. Following the domain name is a "/," and the text that follows that is the *pathway* of the URL—its specific location on the hosting computer within the hierarchy of files and folders.

Figure 11.1

Part A is the resource type; parts B, C, and D make up the domain name, which specifies a particular computer; and parts E and F specify the path name, which locates the resource on that computer.

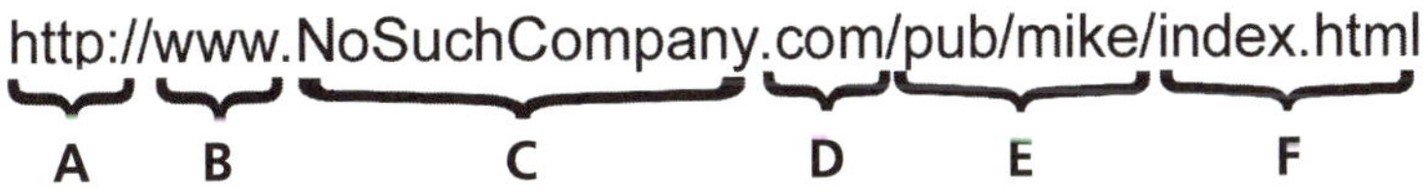

The Components of a Uniform Resource Locator (URL)

A) ***The resource type.*** *The most common one used today is "http://," which refers to a Web site. It is an acronym for hypertext transfer protocol, the standard by which Web pages are transmitted over the Internet. It is increasingly being omitted from printed URLs as understood, as Web addresses become more commonplace.*

B) ***The leading word of the domain name portion of the URL.*** *The "www" word is used to designate a Web server, or a computer that provides information for distribution over the Web. It is not technically part of the domain name.*

C) ***The second-level domain.*** *In this case, it refers to an imaginary company that is operating a Web server. If there were another word between "www" and "NoSuchCompany," it would be considered the third-level domain (remember that "www" is not technically considered a part of the domain name).*

D) ***The top-level domain.*** *This specifies the type of domain—in this case, ".com" designates a commercial enterprise. Other top-level domains include two-letter country codes (mainly used outside of the United States), as well as United States government (.gov), military (.mil), educational (.edu), organizational (.org), and network (.net) domains.*

E) ***The path name*** *(or pathway) that specifies that the file of interest is to be found in a folder called "mike" which is inside a folder called "pub" on the computer specified by the domain name. Note that the computer specified by the domain name can be real (an actual physical computer) or virtual (existing as a subsection of some other computer, which may be unknown to the site visitor).*

F) ***The file name*** *containing the Web page specified by the URL.*

The Domain Name System

The *domain name system* (DNS) requires further explanation. Every host computer connected to the Internet must be identified by a unique code. The code actually used by computers to locate each other is known as the IP (Internet protocol) address, and is a string of four three-digit numbers, separated by periods. However, such a code is not easily remembered by human beings, and is certainly not an easily recognizable "brand name" when the time comes to market a Web site to the Internet community.

Each unique IP address can be converted into a string of words known as a *domain name*. The words are separated by periods, and have specific limitations on length (67 letters) and characters used (no spaces or special symbols such as "@," "#," or "$"). Each domain name consists of two or more words, with the last one being the *top-level domain*. Computers known as "DNS servers" perform the conversion of these words into IP addresses and back again.

The list of registered domain names is a widely distributed database, updated at regular intervals and maintained by any one of a number of regional *registries*, which are accredited entities that perform this function for the Internet community. Accreditation of registries (among other functions) is now performed by a non-profit organization known as ICANN (The Internet Corporation for Assigned Names and Numbers), which has an international board of directors.[1]

Top-Level Domains

The top-level domain in countries outside of the United States is a two-letter code assigned to that country by Internet standards. There is a ".us" country code for the United States, but it is rarely used. Rather, a set of descriptive top-level domains are used in the United States to specify whether the domain is owned, for example, by an educational institution (.edu), a military organization (.mil), or a governmental entity (.gov). The commercial (.com) domain is the most popular, having originally been intended for businesses. However, the term ".com" has become so widespread that is has entered common English usage, and many of these domains are not true commercial organizations. Other domains used in the United States are for networks (.net) and generic organizations (.org). Special verification is necessary to claim some domains (such as .gov, .edu, or .mil), while others may be registered by anyone (such as .com, .org, and .net).

The ICANN is the regulatory body that approves top-level domain names, recommending them for implementation. As of November 2000, seven new top-level domain proposals were selected for further negotiation, prior to approval for registration. These include .coop (nonprofit cooperatives), .museum (museums), .name (individuals), and .pro (doctors, lawyers, and accountants). Among the 40 additional proposals turned down by ICANN was the .health domain, presumably because of the implied content regulation difficulties. The World Health Organization, which sponsored the .health proposal, intends to appeal the ICANN decision as of this writing.

Second-Level Domains and Virtual Addresses

The other parts of the domain name (to the left of the top-level domain) specify the particular computer registered under that name. The label "www" is by convention appended to the front of most Web site domain names, but is not necessary and is not actually a part of the registered domain name. It is used to refer to a computer acting as a Web server. The pathway may be omitted for clarity, in which case the default pathway is assumed—a file named "index.html" at the host site. The resource type "http://" is also assumed, and is typically omitted when the URL is used in print. Furthermore, the "www" and the ".com" are so common that most Web browsers will just assume that they are present if a single word is entered as an address. Therefore, for example, most modern browsers will translate "NoSuchCompany" into http://www.NoSuchCompany.com/index.html if nothing else is specified. In this case, "NoSuchCompany" is the second-level domain.

While every Internet host computer must have a domain name, not every domain name has to refer to a specific computer. Many people and organizations register domain names and then use them to direct traffic to a Web site hosted elsewhere. The domain name is the recognized "brand name" linked to the online resource or business—the actual location of the resource is arbitrary and changeable, and may never be noticed by site visitors. For example, typing the URL "www.Kids-ENT.com" into a Web browser actually refers to a specific folder on a specific computer belonging to a commercial Internet service provider. They rent this space to me, enable me to maintain my Web site files, and provide hosting for the site. A few months ago, I changed from one service provider to another, which changed the actual location of these files. This change was irrelevant to the Internet community, which sees Kids-ENT.com as a constant "brand name." The Kids-ENT.com domain is considered a *virtual* address, meaning that it itself does not refer to an actual computer but rather is (temporarily) linked to a subsection of a real, physical computer.

How Web Pages Are Stored and Delivered

In Figure 11.2, NoSuchCompany, Inc, maintains a computer that it uses as its Web server. This host computer is identified to the other computers on the Internet by the numerical (IP) address "123.456.789.000." However, to allow for easier human recognition, the domain name "NoSuchCompany.com" has been registered as being equivalent to this IP address, and the Web server is given the name www.NoSuchCompany.com by the domain name service (DNS) server computers.

On the Web server, there are a number of folders in hierarchical arrangement, including the one corresponding to my account ("mike"). The "mike" folder is found in the larger "pub" folder, which contains all of the accounts rented out by the company. I could use this account for a number of projects, including the Kids-ENT Web site, which I can maintain in a folder called "ent."

Figure 11.2

An example of how Web pages are stored and delivered.

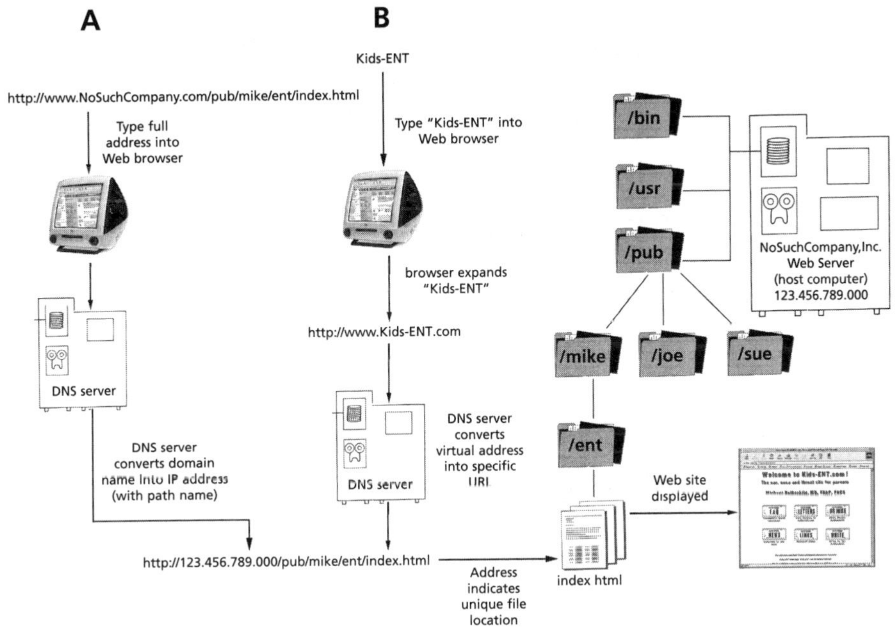

I have independently registered the domain "Kids-ENT.com," and specified that it refer to the specific folder "ent." This is a virtual address because there is no physical computer called "Kids-ENT.com," but rather, it refers to a folder on another computer.

To see this Web site, the visitor can type either the full address into the browser (Path A), or the abbreviated address (Path B). In Path A, the address is passed to a DNS server, which converts it into the IP address and path name. This file is then retrieved, and displayed by the browser as the Kids-ENT Web page. In Path B, the visitor only needs to type in "Kids-ENT" (much easier to remember and print). The browser assumes that this means http://www.Kids-ENT.com, converts it to this full address, and then passes that address to the DNS server. The DNS server again does the appropriate lookup, and determines the unique IP address and path name, displaying the Web page.

The Marketing Value of a Good Domain Name

A good domain name is incredibly valuable, especially if a Web site is to be marketed. In fact, since the term "dot com" has become a part of the English language, almost all domains represented by single words followed by ".com" have been registered. Some of the more valuable ones have become prized properties, registered by speculators hoping to sell them at a higher price. If these prices seem high to you, just remember how much it costs to build brand identity in the world beyond the Internet. Imagine how much it would cost you to buy the rights to the names "Coca Cola" or "Microsoft"!

Prices ($) Recently Paid at Auction for Selected Domain Names

Business.com	*7.5 million*
AsSeenOnTV.com	*5 million*
Loans.com	*3 million*
Wisdom.com	*475,000*
Internet.com	*100,000*

While single English words are generally a part of the public domain, proper names are in some cases considered to be subject to copyright laws, and there have been several court cases regarding domain registration. Some of these have involved legitimate disputes, in which both parties felt that they had a claim to the name, and others have been cases of "cybersquatting," in which a domain name based on a well-known celebrity or trademarked brand has been registered in hopes of reselling it to the "rightful owner" for a profit.

Ideally, you should be able to secure an easy-to-remember domain name that is logically linked to your practice. This is less important (but still a consideration) if you will be primarily using your Web site for established patients. In general, the more specific (and longer) your domain name, the more likely it is to be available. Nothing is to stop you from registering "doctor.com" (except the fact that someone else has already done it). Similarly, "DoctorSmith.com" has been taken. If your name is less common, you may be able to pick up a domain of this type for the usual $35 per year fee. For example, "DoctorWimpleby.com" was still available as of this writing. If your name is Smith and you like the idea of a Web site named "DoctorSmith," you have two choices: make an offer to the owner of "DoctorSmith.com" (a manufacturer of baby care products), or register a variant of the domain name.

Domain name variants can be made by either choosing the ".net" or ".org" versions of the name, or by adding something to the name that does not detract too much from its brevity or meaning (eg, "DoctorSmithOnline.com"). Given the fact that ".com" is the default assumption by most Web browsers, you should always try to secure a ".com" version if at all possible. Finally, do not be reluctant to register multiple versions of a domain name if you are planning an aggressive marketing campaign. Thirty-five dollars a year isn't much in the scheme of things, and having a number of variants can mean capturing visitors who might go elsewhere. Many large businesses will register plural versions of their domain names or common misspellings, both to increase traffic at their sites and to prevent mischievous individuals from publishing inappropriate material under their brand.

If you are contemplating an online presence at all, and you have a unique practice name that you would like to secure as a domain name, then by all means register the domain at once. Every 5 seconds, a new domain is registered, and you never know when yours will be taken. You can secure the domain without having a Web site or even a place to store it—the registry itself can "park" the domain for you (for a nominal fee) until you are ready to launch a Web site.

If you have a domain in which a single word is made up from more than one word, it may not be immediately apparent what your domain name represents. For example, I chose "Kids-ENT.com" to reflect my pediatric otolaryngology practice. I also registered the same name without the dash, and had this version—"kidsent.com"—simply linked to the main site. The version with the dash is better for printing (such as on letterhead or business cards). On the other hand, I often give someone the name of the Web site verbally. I can simply say "check out Kids ENT dot com," and even if they omit the dash when remembering it later, they will still reach the correct site. Web sites are usually case insensitive, so feel free to use interspersed capitals to improve readability: "KidsENT.com" is easier to understand in print than "kidsent.com."

Some organizations that provide Web site space to physicians will enable you to register as a subdomain or a higher-level domain on their server. There is generally no charge for this, and this technique is frequently found on the "Wizard" sites discussed in Chapter 6. For example, Medem and Salu.net add a third-level domain in front of their own (ie, www.Kids-ENT.yourmd.com and www.DoctorMike.salu.net), while Medscape provides for a subdomain (doctor.medscape.com/kidsent). While this does allow for some degree of practice brand recognition, it is still preferable to have your own unique domain name for marketing purposes.

Finally, some companies have taken to "exploiting" the unique two-letter country codes that identify Web sites outside of the United States. Although a server must be in a given country to use that top-level domain, entrepreneurs have realized that some country codes are more recognizable than others, and have marketing value (Figure 11.3). The eastern European country of Moldova does not have a large Internet industry, but it has luckily been assigned the country code ".md." While this has no special meaning in the native language, it obviously has great appeal for American physicians. Many doctors have paid a significant premium to register a domain such as "DoctorSmith.MD" on a Moldovan server, and then have the domain redirect the visitor to a medical Web site. Hopefully, a portion of those revenues will find their way to the hosting countries in this scheme of "Internet colonialism"!

Figure 11.3

Countries with top-level domain names that are appealing from a marketing point of view.

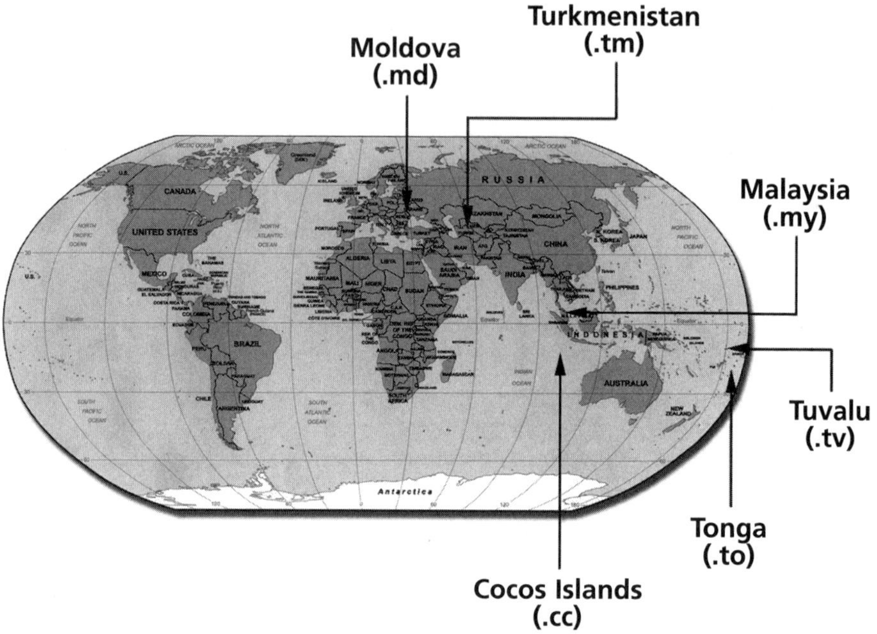

Hosting

Once you have registered your domain name and constructed your Web site, the pages must be placed on a Web server. There are several options for this hosting service. Of course, it is important that the computer on which your pages reside is reliable and has a stable connection to the Internet. Hosting can cost thousands of dollars a month in the case of companies that require significant bandwidth. Usually, however, bandwidth is not an issue for medical practice sites, as most will not generate extremely heavy traffic or serve high-volume data streams (such as video). It would be extremely uncommon for a practice to need a high-capacity Internet link for its public Web site.

If you have contracted with a full-service Web design company, they will probably offer you a hosting contract. This is usually fairly expensive, but may include continual site maintenance and ongoing consultation. Be sure not to purchase any services that you do not need, as hosting can be done with minimal costs, as discussed below. If you have a low-cost alternative for hosting, you may be able to negotiate with the company so that you pay for maintenance only (if you require even that). Most commercial Internet service providers (such as the ones that enable you to connect from your home) will provide a certain amount of Web server space with their standard dial-up accounts. This is usually enough for the typical practice site. My current ISP charges about $30 a month for a package including Internet access, two e-mail accounts, and 8 megabytes of Web server space. Previously, I hosted the Kids-ENT site for $10 a month with a company that provided server space only.

If your practice's Internet access is "always on," as is the case with newer services such as digital subscriber lines (DSL) or cable modems, you can actually host the site from any computer in your office (assuming that this is acceptable to your service provider). However, this requires that the computer be running 24 hours a day. It also involves having someone always available to attend to any unanticipated problems such as crashes, and firewall software to prevent unauthorized access ("hacking") from outside. The advantages of this are that your Web server space is only limited by the space on your hard drive, and that no further monthly hosting costs are involved. Remember, though, that the costs of such continual access will be higher, and that most Web sites for individual practices do not require more than a few megabytes of storage space. Furthermore, the less expensive versions of DSL service are asymmetric, meaning that the capacity to send information from your computer *to* the Internet is considerably less than the capacity to retrieve information *from* the Internet. Most businesses that host their own Web sites using DSL opt for the more expensive symmetric version of the service, which provides for equal capacity in both directions.

Frequently, hosting can be arranged through an organization or educational entity with which you have a relationship. This is the case with the wizard sites described earlier in this chapter and in Chapter 6, and may be possible if you have an academic affiliation. Keep in mind the importance of reliability and performance, however. If a Web server is frequently inoperable or slow, it will make visiting your site a frustrating experience.

Endnote

1. The Internet Corporation for Assigned Names and Numbers Web site. Available at: www.icann.org.

Chapter 12
Web Site Promotion

"If a tree falls in the forest and there is no one there to hear it, does it make a sound?"

Anonymous

Just like the tree in the forest, even the best Web site will have no impact unless someone comes to visit. In order to market your practice on the Internet, you must market your Web site as well. For sites that are primarily intended for your established patients or new patients referred through traditional routes, it is enough to provide each person with the site URL printed on, for example, a business card or letterhead. Cards specifically oriented toward the site can be given out in addition to your conventional business cards, and included in letters sent to referring physicians (Figure 12.1).

Figure 12.1

Two business cards incorporating the Kids-ENT.com URL. (A) The conventional business card. The URL is listed below the hospital faculty page. (B) A card oriented toward the Web site. Note the use of a separate e-mail address associated with the Kids-ENT domain (arrow). This address is set up to automatically forward mail to the more frequently checked mailbox.

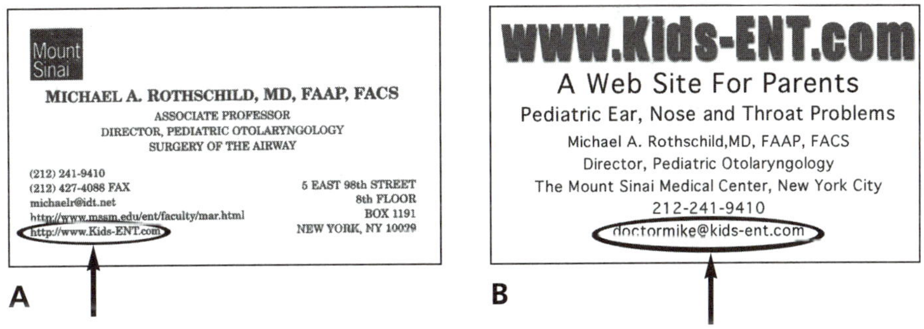

In general, it is usually best to defer aggressive marketing of your Web site until you have registered your own domain name. For example, I have www.Kids-ENT.com printed on my letterhead and business cards, but I did not have the original URL printed up in the same way (which was something like http://www.NoSuchCompany.com/Kids-ENT/index.html). Although most doctors who are serious about marketing their practices online will sooner or later register a unique and catchy domain name, many start out with a preliminary Web site URL based on an academic server or a commercial site creation enterprise. It is common for this URL to change, because you eventually get your own domain name, or you switch hosting services, or the host decides to rearrange its directory structure. Although you may be able to arrange for the old URL to point to your new site, this may not be possible once you stop doing business with your former host. The best approach is to secure the domain name first (even before building the Web site), and then use it for marketing purposes. (See Chapter 11 for more information on registering a domain name.)

If you plan on using the site to capture new business, or would like to provide medical information to the Internet community at large, you will need to ensure that your site is easy to find online. Although some people will use techniques such as asking visitors to bookmark your site, or mentioning the name of the site on an Internet discussion forum, online site marketing is primarily done through specialized Web resources known as *search engines* and *directories*—the main way Web users find new sites.

Search Engines

A search engine is an Internet resource that returns a list of Web sites in response to the user submitting one or more keywords or search terms. Typically, these engines are composed of three components: a program that combs the Internet for information about Web sites (called the "spider" or "crawler"); a large database (or index) of this information assembled by the spider; and a mechanism for selecting and ranking sites from the database based on the search terms. The higher the search engine ranks your page, the better, as few Web users will look past the first page or two of search results.

As of mid-2000, the publicly indexable Web consists of over a billion individual Web pages! A study published in 1999 estimated approximately 800 million pages, and determined that none of the search engine databases had indexed more than 16% of these, a proportion that had been dropping as the Web in general expanded in the last years of the 20th century.[1] More recently, however, the number of indexed pages has risen, as has the indexed percentage of the Web as a whole. Some engines claim to have close to 100% of the indexable Web in their database (Figure 12.2).[2] However, bigger is not always better. In many situations, a directed search of a smaller database may return more useful sites than a broad search of a large percentage of the Web (which tends to return many irrelevant pages).

Figure 12.2

Web site from the Google search engine (www.google.com), which claims to index over a billion pages (close to all of those on the publicly indexable Web).

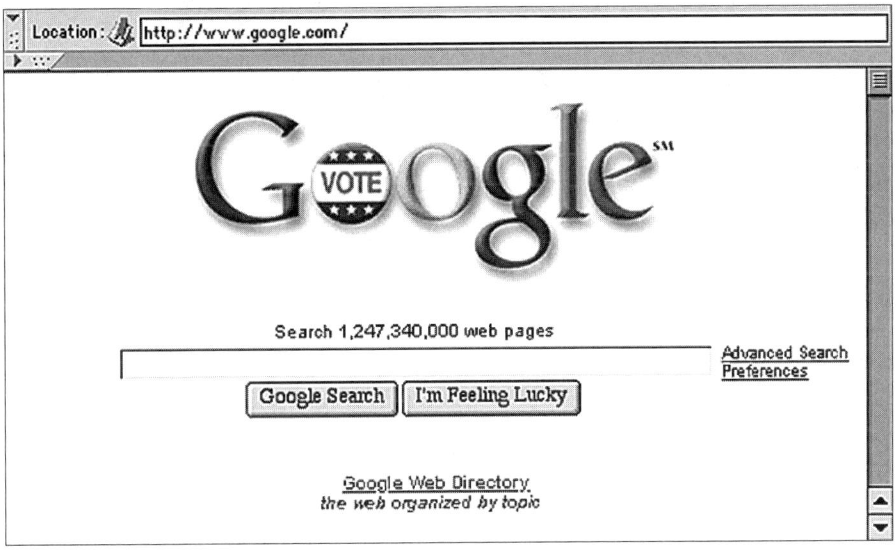

There are a number of popular search engines, and each has a different approach to ranking. In order to enhance the rank of your site, it is important to know something about ranking mechanisms. Unfortunately, this can be a moving target as the companies that operate these engines are constantly modifying their protocols. These companies are selling a service, and can only retain a customer base if their engines consistently produce useful lists of relevant links in answer to any request. Table 12.1 provides a listing of the major search engines on the Web today.

Table 12.1

Comparison of Major Search Engines, as of Mid-2000

Engine	Deep crawl*?	Link popularity boosts depth of crawl?	META tag boosts rank?	Instant indexing**?	Frames?	Number of pages indexed (millions as of 6/00[2])	Strengths
AltaVista	+	—	—	+	+	350	Large, comprehensive, powerful search commands
Excite	+	—	—	—	—	250	Concept searching feature, helps narrow search
Fast Search	+	—	—	—	+	575	Large database
Go (Infoseek)	—	—	+	—	—	50	Good search algorithm and portal features
Google	+	—	—	—	+	560	Very large, heavily weighted toward link popularity. Actually indexes a further 500 million pages beyond those visited by the spider, based on inference from links
Inktomi	+	+	+	—	—	500	Index behind many other search tools, not directly searchable
Northern Light	+	—	—	—	+	265	Classification feature, special (nonpublic) content

** The term "deep crawl" refers to the spider's ability to index beyond the top-level page of a Web site.*

*** An engine that features "instant indexing" will rapidly reflect changes in a Web site (within days rather than the usual months).*

In the early days of the Web, search ranking was dependent on the number of times a search term appeared on a page. Therefore, you could make your site rise to the top by including multiple copies of relevant keywords on your Web pages in text that was not visibly displayed. For example, if I were to place the word "otitis" 50 times in small white text on a white background at the bottom of my page, my site might be ranked above a site that only used the word 10 times, and appear ahead of that site when someone typed "otitis" into the search window. This approach ("keyword stuffing") is now frowned upon and may actually cause your site to be downgraded.

Another formerly employed technique similar to keyword stuffing was the inclusion of common but irrelevant search terms (such as "money," "sex," or "Internet") to make your site appear frequently, in hopes of obtaining free advertising to people doing general searches. Again, this practice is not appropriate and may result in penalization by the ranking mechanism of modern search engines.

Search engines assemble their databases from the spider program's reading of Web sites. Not every spider will read all of the text contained on your pages—some will only read and index the first few words or paragraphs. However, certain parts of a Web page are more likely to be read and indexed, and should be carefully assembled with this in mind. The title of the page should not only stand alone as a descriptive phrase, but should contain as many keywords as possible that pertain to the content, as spiders will certainly index the title. Text contained inside a portion of the page delimited by "Meta" tags is not displayed in a browser, but serves as a placeholder for keywords that describe the site and aid in indexing by the engine. Up to 1000 characters (including spaces and commas) can be included in this section. Finally, "Alt" tags should be employed as well. "Alt" stands for alternative, and is appended to an image so that a browser that does not display pictures (such as those used by patients with limited vision) will be able to put a descriptive phrase in the image's place, which can be enlarged or read aloud by speech synthesizing software. Since a search engine cannot index a picture, having descriptive text here is important to aid the engine in thoroughly indexing your site. It is important to keep all of this text up to date, because a site that has been recently updated will often be ranked higher than a "cobweb" site.

Frames are particularly troublesome when it comes to search engines. Apart from the reasons mentioned in Chapter 7, another reason to avoid frames is that some engines will not be able to index text within a frame, or will return links that lead to isolated frames taken out of the intended context.

Lately, link popularity has become a major consideration in ranking. Engines assume that the more sites that link to yours, the more popular your site must be. In order to evaluate your site's popularity as a target of links, you can either review the logs from your host computer (which may summarize the addresses of all sites leading to yours), or use a search engine. To do the latter, just type "link:" followed by your domain name (omitting the "www." at the front) into the search window at AltaVista or Infoseek (Figure 12.3). Anything that you can do to get other sites to link to yours will therefore help improve your ranking by many search engines. Directly contacting the Webmasters of health-related Web sites and making a case for the usefulness of your content can result in your being added to a list of links. Reciprocal linking arrangements, in which you link to someone's site in exchange for their linking to yours, are common. "Webrings" are a similar concept, in which sites on a common topic are linked sequentially, enabling the visitor to "tour the Internet" in a specific field by going from one site to the next.

Figure 12.3

Results of a link search on the Kids-ENT domain.

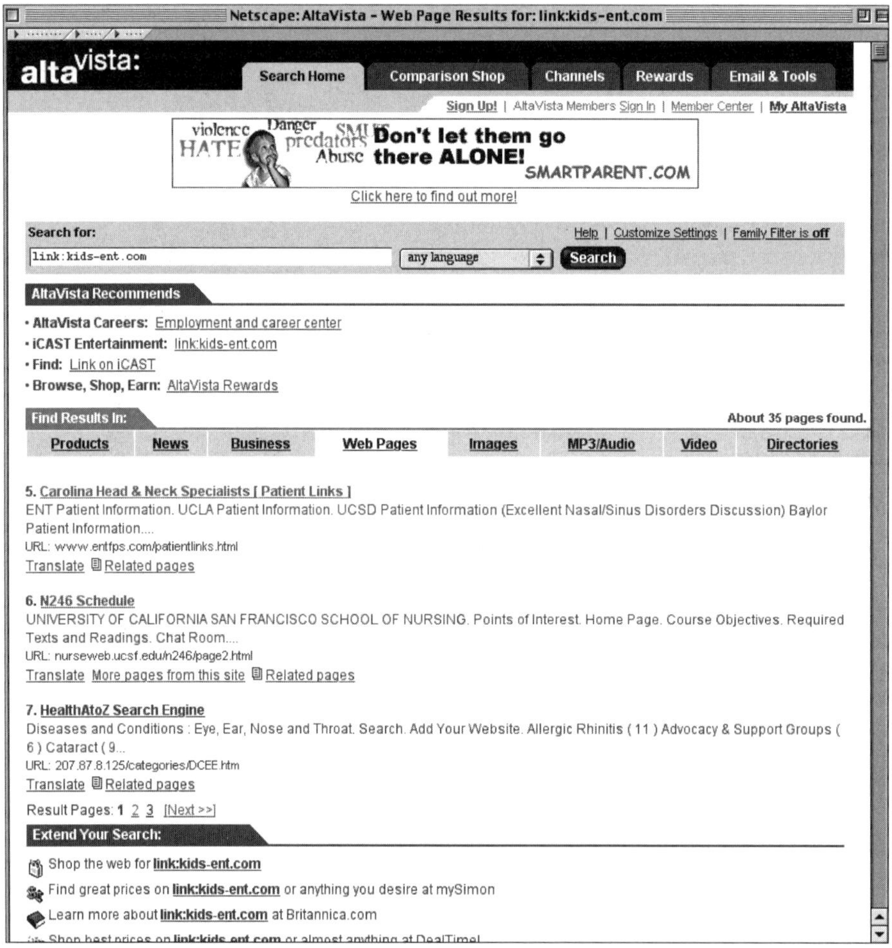

Another recent trend in search engines is the use of "collaborative filtering." In this case, different ranking mechanisms are used for each user, based on information supplied by the user of his or her likes, dislikes, and other preferences. The search of the index is modified by the profile generated about that user. Ideally, this should generate more relevant search results.

Directories

The other main type of Internet search tool is the directory. Unlike a search engine, a directory is complied by human reviewers who evaluate specific sites, determine whether they are worthy of being listed, categorized them by content, and, in some cases, write capsule reviews. This has the advantage of excluding the thousands of irrelevant links that may be returned by a search engine in response to a general query. However, directories are limited by their personnel resources, and new sites may take quite a while to get listed. For example, Open Directory (www.dmoz.org) is reported to receive 250 submissions per hour.

A directory is more useful when a few high-quality sites are needed in a very broad field, while a search engine would be better for finding sites on a very specific or unusual topic. Because directories can only list sites that they have reviewed, and can only review sites that they know about, it may be necessary to submit your Web site for review. Each directory has a protocol for site submission. When your practice Web site is ready for public launching, it should be submitted to the more popular general directories, as well as those focusing on health-related resources.

It is important to recognize that the directory editors in a particular field may be overwhelmed and you will have to be helpful in providing as much information as possible. Alternatively, an automated submission service can prepare an "application" for a large number of directories, usually for a small fee. While saving some time, this approach may actually be less effective than taking the time to tailor your appeal to the largest directories and ignoring the less influential ones. Getting your site listed on a major directory will probably result in more traffic than getting listed on a large number of minor directories. To put this in perspective, an estimated 30% of all traffic to sites engaging in online commerce is referred through Yahoo! (www.yahoo.com).

In order to obtain a Yahoo! listing (which is extremely valuable in the field of online marketing), certain techniques may help. It is important to be specific as to which subcategory would be appropriate for your site. This speeds the process and enhances your chances, as you are competing in a smaller arena. Do not suggest that your interventional cardiology group be listed under "health," but rather find the exact specialty category that would be the best fit. Provide information as to the physical location of your practice, as some Yahoo! users might look for a doctor by first searching in the regional category that corresponds to their home.

Hybrids and Paid Listings

Many companies providing Web searching capabilities have now expanded their offerings to provide a hybrid of a directory service and a search engine (see Table 12.2). This enables the user to draw on the strength of both approaches, picking up sites from a vast engine database while first being offered hand-selected, high-quality sites based on the same keywords. A common arrangement is for a search engine site to supplement its results with directory entries (as AltaVista does with the Open Directory project). Alternatively, a directory might use a search engine as a backup if no specific hand-picked entry was found for a given search. Figure 12.4 summarizes the relationships between search engines, directories, and hybrids. Some of these hybrid services are presented as Web "portals," which are single sites that combine the search tool with other frequently requested content (such as weather, news, sports information, and stock quotes).

Figure 12.4

Diagram showing the mechanism of search engines, directories, and hybrid sites. Note that these features change fairly rapidly.

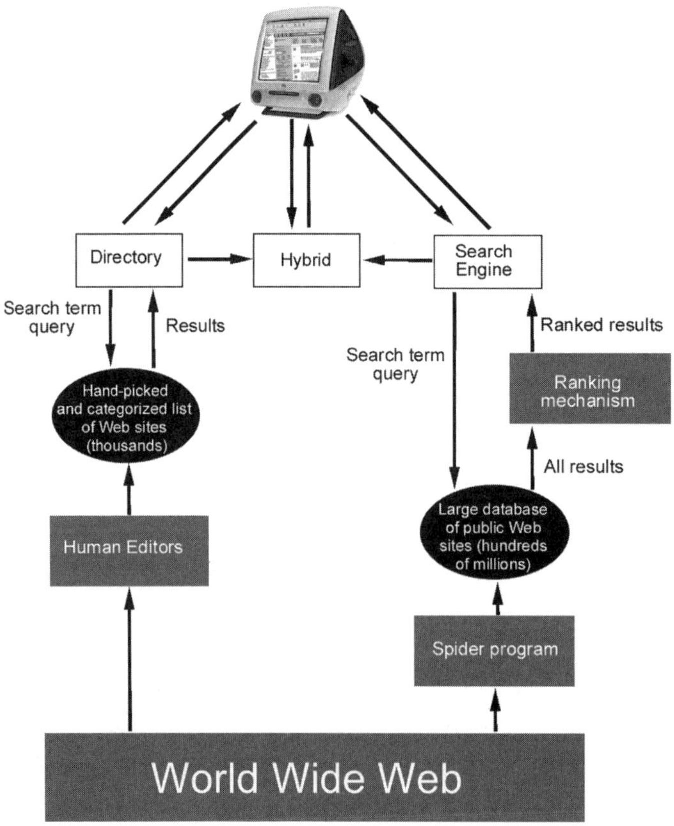

Table 12.2

A Comparison of the Popular Web Directories and Engine/Directory Hybrids (as of mid-2000)

Yahoo	By far the largest and most influential, with over 150 editors and over 1 million hand-picked sites. Directory links are supplemented by search engine results from Google (formerly from Inktomi).
Lycos	Formerly a search engine, now providing directory results from the Open Directory project.
Open Directory	A volunteer project, now owned by Netscape but providing its entries to a number of other sites through open licensing (such as Netscape, Lycos, AOL Search, AltaVista, and HotBot).
LookSmart	Provides entries to MSN search, Excite, and its own site. Supplements directory searches with Inktomi results.
MSN Search	Microsoft product providing directory entries from LookSmart and engine results from Inktomi
Netscape Search	Directory entries from Open Directory, as well as the Netscape database. Supplements directory searches with Google results.
AOL Search	Has both an internal version (listing America Online content) and an external version (listing only Web content). Directory entries from Open Directory, with supplementary search engine results from Inktomi.
Snap	A directory backed by CNET and NBC. Supplements its listings with Inktomi results.
Go	Owned by Disney. Provides directory services as well as search engine results from the acquired Infoseek engine.

A new approach to listing and ranking provides an additional revenue stream to the directory company. Search tools such as GoTo.com auction off ranking positions to advertisers, who pay a certain referral fee for each person who finds their site this way. After all of the paid advertisers have been listed (in descending order of their bid prices, with the referral fee listed), a general search engine result list is displayed. One problem with this is that the judgment of a category editor—who functions to rate sites and only list the best—is replaced by the free market. However, for some types of niche sales markets, this may be appropriate, enabling a small businessman in a very specific business (eg, antique medical books) to compete with a giant (such as Amazon.com) without paying huge fees for prominent banner ads or other promotion. The small business does not pay for marketing to the general Internet community, which is likely to have a low yield—but spends its scarce advertising dollars on the few people who have expressed an interest in their product.

This approach seems less useful in the medical community, where patients expect unbiased recommendations regarding quality Web sites. However, there are some parallels to conventional practice marketing, such as Yellow Page ads, where the practices that spend more are likely to see more referrals. The classic example of this is a full fee-for-service cosmetic surgery group. Practices that realize lesser returns for each new patient would be less inclined to pay for ranking on a search engine. To illustrate this point, a GoTo.com search for "plastic surgery" revealed 48 paid placement sites (with referral fees paid to the site ranging from $0.01 to $1.05), followed by a standard search engine list based on this phrase (provided by Inktomi). When the term "pediatrics" was used, only 13 paid sites were returned (at $0.01 to $0.41), and the phrase "pediatric otolaryngology" did not return any paid sites at all (likely due in part to the small size of the subspecialty).

Search engine ranking strategies and index design continue to evolve at a rapid pace. At this point, it requires an ongoing interest in the field to keep up with all of the latest developments in ranking mechanisms. This is one of the reasons why it might be helpful to use a professional Web design company that provides site marketing as one of its services. If you are doing the marketing yourself, it pays to monitor new developments through one of the many Web sites devoted to this particular industry, such as Danny Sullivan's Search Engine Watch (www.searchenginewatch.com) shown in Figure 12.5.[2]

Figure 12.5

The Search Engine Watch Web site (www.searchenginewatch.com), which provides up-to-date information about strategies used in search engine design, as well as a basic understanding of the issues involved in using and constructing Web search tools.[2] (Reprinted with permission from http://www.internet.com. Copyright © 2001 internet.com Corporation.)

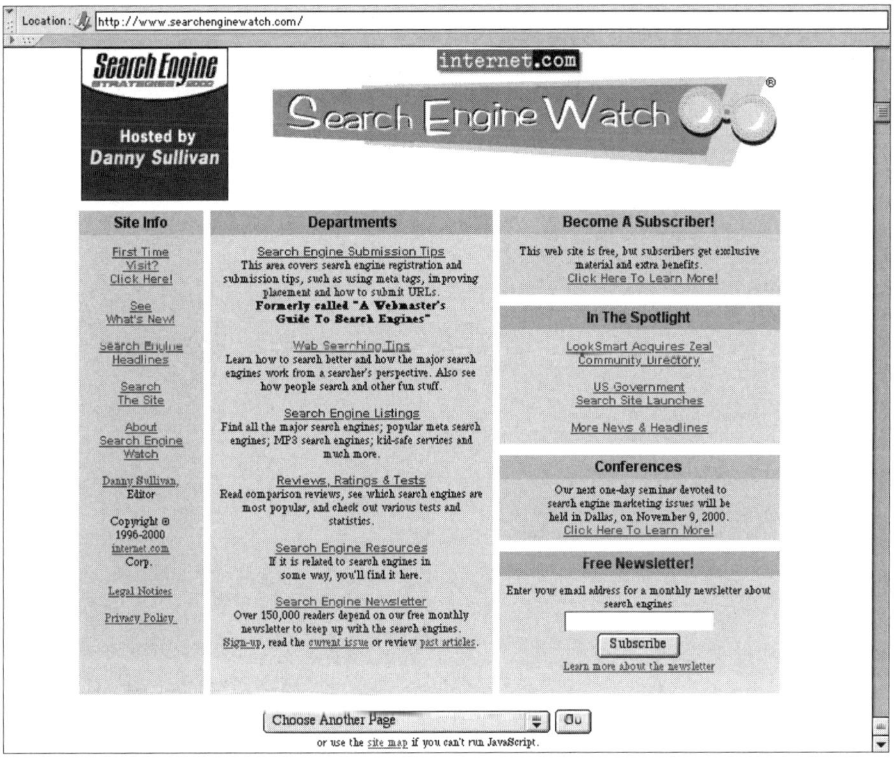

As was mentioned earlier, certain search engines will downgrade sites that have not recently been updated. While good content is important, content that is both of high quality *and current* is especially valuable on the medical Internet. In the next chapter, we will therefore turn to the important topic of site maintenance.

Endnotes

1. Lawrence S, Giles CL. Accessibility of information on the web. *Nature*. 1999;400:107-109.
2. Search Engine Watch Web site. Available at: www.searchenginewatch.com.

Chapter 13
Ongoing Web Site Maintenance and Monitoring

"I know half the money I spend on advertising is wasted, but I can never find out which half."

Leo Burnett (1891-1971), advertising executive

Once your site has been created, carefully checked, hosted, and marketed, there is a tendency to forget about it for a while. After all, one of the advantages of a Web site is that it provides information continually without requiring any human attention. While this is true, it is always important to keep your site as current as possible. Furthermore, as with any marketing campaign, it is necessary to assess the value received for the money spent, to help budget for future expenditures.

Patients often choose physicians based on their health plan participation, and in many practices, participation varies with time. A new patient who calls for an appointment or an established patient who makes a special trip to your office based on your plan participation as listed on the Web site will not be happy if this information is out of date. Furthermore, supplementary information on office staff, new partners, and clinic hours should be meticulously kept current, especially as more and more people come to rely on the Web as a primary information resource. Finally, as was mentioned in Chapter 12, search engines may downgrade a Web site that has not been recently updated.

However you assemble your site, it is important that you have ready access to the pages for regular updates. If you have an ongoing consulting relationship with your Web design firm, they certainly can make minor changes in content. However, this should be a trivial task, and you should not be charged much for the service. Similarly, it is not wise to pay a large monthly "maintenance" fee to a Web company if the only changes to be made are minor text editing. You should own the code of the Web site you purchased and be able to make such minor changes yourself if you feel capable. Larger additions (such as a profile page for a new partner, or changes in the layout) might be done for a fee negotiated on a case-by-case basis. Be sure that any Web site code you purchase is well-documented so that it can be maintained even if you are no longer doing business with the original author. Also, it should be "portable," so that it can be moved from computer to computer without requiring any recoding.

Medical content will require intermittent maintenance as well. Any clinical information should reflect the current state of your practice and the medical literature as well as possible. Furthermore, occasional inclusion of new content will make visitors more likely to return to your site. Affiliation with a medical society or corporate content service may allow for regular automatic updating with medical news feeds. Be sure that any external links remain current, as you will have no notice if one of your suggested Internet resources suddenly shuts down. This will minimize "dead links," which make your site seem unprofessional and stagnant.

A helpful resource in keeping your site up to date is the statistics page provided by your Web hosting entity. Almost all hosts provide extensive information regarding site traffic, including the number of times each page on the site was accessed, the traffic at various dates and times, and the domains and Web sites from which your visitors have arrived. This can be useful in planning content additions or in directing your site marketing efforts.

For example, suppose that your dermatology practice provides information about skin care online, and you determine that the pages on sun exposure are accessed much more frequently than the other pages. In this case, you might consider expanding this section of the site with more content, photographs, and external links. Similarly, if you determine that several search engines and directories are providing you with a large number of referrals, but, for instance, Yahoo! is not, you might want to direct your site marketing efforts toward Yahoo! to enhance your traffic.

Examination of the Kids-ENT.com statistics for last month demonstrated that search terms related to the ear were almost 10 times as likely to be used in finding the site than terms related to the tonsils. This suggests that there may be more interest in ear disease among people searching the Web for health information than in tonsillar disease, and I might want to add more resources about ear infections and hearing loss. This is corroborated by a report that indicates that the ear pages are accessed much more often than the pages related to tonsillitis or sinusitis. I can also determine that while the vast majority of traffic comes from Internet host computers in the United States (as expected), almost 6% comes from the United Kingdom and Canada, followed by 1.5% from New Zealand. The list of countries accessing the Kids-ENT site continues, providing me with the knowledge that in the last month I have received, among others, 115 visitors from Malaysia, 42 from Macedonia, 14 from Latvia, and seven from Luxembourg.

Perhaps the most important data for any marketing effort is the efficacy of the campaign to justify its expense. Web sites are somewhat different from other forms of mass media advertising—the initial development costs are a much greater percentage of the total expenditures than in, for example, print ads or television commercials (where ongoing costs are high). Furthermore, there are many intangible benefits of enhancing doctor-patient communication, which may not be reflected in the "bottom line." However, it will still be useful to have a general estimate of the Web site's impact on patient visits, especially if you are contemplating an expensive, custom-built site.

The return-on-investment figure may be difficult to accurately assess in this situation, as patients may be referred to the office in multiple ways. Some may receive a recommendation through conventional channels (such as word of mouth, or their primary care physician), and then decide to make an appointment after visiting your site. Others may have found you through the Internet, but will not volunteer this information even if asked. My feeling is that as the costs of medical practice Web sites continue to drop, and more and more practices develop them, this analysis will be increasingly less important. After all, no one spends much time calculating the return on investment of a fax machine. Rather, this is just considered one of the many small costs of running a modern medical practice.

In this book, we have considered the reasons to maintain an online presence for your medical practice, and reviewed some of the basic steps necessary in planning and executing an Internet marketing effort. Any book about the Internet is almost certainly out of date by the time it appears in print, as the online world continues to develop new trends, features, and communities. However, I hope that the points that have been made here are general enough to be useful to physicians who are just venturing into the online world, as well as to those who have developed Web sites and seek to improve them. As always, I am happy to respond as best I can to specific e-mail inquiries about this topic.

Michael Rothschild, MD
DoctorMike@Kids-ENT.com

Appendix A
Common Errors in Web Site Creation

This appendix provides a list of some of the more common errors encountered in the creation of a Web site. Even if you have outsourced the development of your online presence, familiarity with these points will be useful. Many sites created by professional Web designers contain flaws such as these, which should be corrected before the site is launched, and certainly considered in the early stages of authoring. Remember, your Web site reflects your practice and your professional image—you are ultimately responsible for its quality.

Layout Errors

- Not enough early consideration to site architecture
- Overuse or misuse of frames
- Inconsistent or confusing internal navigation
- Lack of navigation buttons on each page
- Points to click for links not clearly indicated
- Dead-end links within the site
- Very long pages of text (should be divided up into subpages)

Design Errors

- Use of fonts that reduce readability
- Use of fonts that are not universally available
- Too many different fonts and/or text colors
- Nonstandard color codes for links
- Distracting background
- Problems with font/background combinations
- Overuse of text styles (eg, bold, italic)
- Overuse or misuse of multimedia and other features (eg, Java applets, sound, animation, video)
- Inconsistent appearance on different browsers
- Requiring the use of special software to view content without providing a simple alternative, and/or a text-only version

Image Errors

- Large graphics
- Poor-quality graphics
- Unnecessary overuse of graphics
- Inadequate graphics (too much text)
- Using GIF instead of JPEG for photographs
- Using JPEG instead of GIF for straight-edged images with few colors
- Nonoptimized graphics (wasted resolution, color depth or physical size)

Content Errors

- Content incomplete at launch (ie, "under construction" sites)
- Inappropriate, dead, or outdated external links
- Inappropriate medical content (noncompliant with guidelines)
- Copied and unattributed content (plagiarism)
- Misappropriated proprietary content (copyright violation)
- Typographical and spelling errors
- Level of content inappropriate for the intended reader

Management Errors

- Overpaid designer/consultant/Webmaster
- Underpaid designer/consultant/Webmaster
- Excessive ongoing costs (eg, hosting, consulting)
- No ownership of Web site code
- Code is not well documented
- Code is not portable
- Lack of a good domain name
- Inability to make minor changes without incurring further costs
- Inadequate site marketing
- Inadequate use of <META>, <TITLE>, and <ALT> tags for keywords
- Lack of usage statistics
- Poor content maintenance

Appendix B
Medem: Your Practice Online

In chapter 6, the various options available to create a practice Web site were discussed. One of the options mentioned was the use of a "wizard"—an online program provided by a sponsoring organization that enables a physician to quickly develop a Web site based on a series of menu driven selections. *Your Practice Online* is one such program.

Your Practice Online is sponsored by Medem, a corporation that manages online content for the American Medical Association and a number of other national and regional medical societies. Web sites are built and hosted using this system free of charge to members of the AMA or any of the other sponsoring organizations. In addition to site creation tools, Medem provides access to a large library of proprietary content for incorporation into the site (such as disease-specific patient education materials). Furthermore, dynamic content in the form of medical news services are available. This ensures that sites created through this program are continually updated without the need for continual revision by the physician. Original content created by the physician (such as brochure text, patient instructions, CVs, and articles) may also be incorporated into a Medem Web site.

For more information about Medem and *Your Practice Online*, see www.yourpracticeonline.com or call 877 926-3336.

Glossary

ADSL — See *DSL*.

Applet — A small program written in the *Java* language that is downloaded from a *Web site* and runs on the site visitor's computer.

ARPANet — Advanced Research Projects Agency Network. The original network project launched by the US Department of Defense in the 1960s that developed into the *Internet*.

ASP — 1) Application Service Provider. A company that enables you to use a specific software package, generally over the Internet, on a rental basis.

2) Active Server Page: A *Web page* containing within its *HTML* code a small script (a type of program) which is processed on a Microsoft *Web server*, generating a custom-made page based on the user's input. This custom page is then displayed for the user. Similar to a common gateway interface *(CGI)* application.

Bandwidth — A term referring to the carrying capacity (speed) of a given *Internet* (or other network) connection. Bandwidth is measured in *bits* per second (*Bps*). There are a number of options for Internet connections—the actual bandwidth achieved depends on a variety of factors such as general network congestion and how many people are sharing a given line.

Banner Ad — A small, rectangular advertisement that appears on many *Web pages*. The sponsor of the ad usually pays for placement on a popular *Web site*, and then pays an additional fee for each "clickthrough"—every time someone clicks on the banner and is transported to the sponsor's *Web site*.

Baud Rate — An older term, referring to the number of times a signal changes in value each second. While often used interchangeably with *Bps*, this is not technically correct and may be inaccurate.

Biometrics — The science of measuring and analyzing biological systems. In the field of medical informatics, the term is frequently used to refer to devices that validate identity by scanning fingerprints, retinal blood vessels, or voice patterns. This may be helpful in authenticating users before access to sensitive information is granted.

Bit — A one or a zero, the smallest unit of digital data. Generally, it takes 8 bits to make up one computer letter, number or other character (*byte*). *Bandwidth* is measured in the number of bits carried per second (*Bps*).

Broadband — A high-speed (high-capacity) link to the Internet. Technically, broadband simply means that the link can carry more than one signal at the same time (as in cable television). In common usage, the term is often applied to applications that require significant *bandwidth*, such as video or high-quality audio transmission.

Browser — A program used to view pages on the *World Wide Web*, as well as to coordinate a variety of other helper programs that do things such as playing sound files, displaying animation, or delivering video.

Bps — *Bits* per second. A measure of *bandwidth*.

Byte — A single digital character (eg, a letter or a number), usually made up of 8 *bits*.

Cable Modem — A device that allows for the use of television cable to provide high-speed *Internet* access, up to around 1 to 2 million *Bps* for downloading, and about 128,000 Bps for uploading. The cable going into a given neighborhood is shared, so that an individual user's *bandwidth* may drop during popular times of *Internet* usage.

CGI — Common gateway interface. A standard way of passing information from a *Web site* user to a program maintained on the *server* (the CGI application), which then generates a result or action that is then sent back to the user. CGI applications can be written in any number of programming languages, but the common ones used for this purpose are C, C++, Java, and PERL. See *ASP*.

Chat — Real-time, text-based communication over the *Internet*, accessed through *Web sites* or other (non-Web) chat software. Users can converse in common areas (chat rooms) on topics of common interest. Mainly used for socializing, but chat-type applications have been used for business and medical teleconferencing as well.

Client — A software program that interacts with a *server* to obtain data. In common usage, the term also has been applied to an individual Web user's personal computer. A *browser* is a type of client software, obtaining *Web pages* from a *server.*

Cobweb Site — A pejorative term referring to a *Web site* that has not been updated in a long time.

Color Depth — The number of different colors that can be represented in an image. Usually given as the number of bits, referring to the binary number used to specify the color of each pixel. Thus, 3-bit color depth would allow for 8 (2 to the 3rd power) different colors and 8-bit color would allow for 256 colors (2 to the 8th power). Sixteen-bit color (65,536 colors) and 24-bit "full color" (16 million colors) are hard to distinguish visually on a computer screen. Black-and-white images are also labeled by color depth, referring to the number of shades of gray. The greater the color depth, the larger the file size.

Cookie — A small file sent by a *Web site* to the visitor's computer, which is then stored in a designated location. The next time the user visits the same site, the cookie can provide information back to the site. This can be innocuous or even beneficial—for instance, when storing registration numbers or account names to provide easier access to sites that are repeatedly visited. Of course, there is always some concern about having anything written onto your computer, and also about the possibility of someone using the information about your Web *surfing* habits inappropriately. Most browsers will allow you to refuse cookies or delete them later.

Crawler — See *Spider.*

DHTML — Dynamic HTML. A more recent version of HTML, with improvements in Web design capabilities.

Dial-up — A type of Internet connection in which the telephone is used to transmit data as a rapidly changing sound signal through a *modem* at each end of the connection. This has been the most common method of *Internet* access for most homes, but is slowly being replaced by faster options such as *cable modems* and *DSL.* The maximum dial-up bandwidth at present is around 56,000 *Bps.*

Directory — A database of *Web sites*, selected by human editors and category experts. Directories can be searched by keywords. The most popular directory as of this writing is Yahoo! (www.yahoo.com).

DNS — Domain name system (or service). A database of Internet addresses, in which unique numerical *IP addresses* are linked to corresponding *domain names*. This database is distributed to multiple computers across the Internet, in the form of DNS *servers*. In this way, an easily remembered *domain name* can be used to specify a location on the *Internet*, and the regularly updated DNS database will ensure that the correct address is used for data transfer.

Domain Name — A series of two or more words separated by periods, which refers to a unique location on the *Internet*. The word furthest to the right is the top-level domain. This refers to the country of registration of the computer being identified (outside the United States), or to the type of computer (commercial, governmental, educational, and so on). A computer known as a *DNS server* converts between the domain name and the actual *IP address.*

Download — The transfer of information from a *host* computer to a *client* system, typically a personal computer of some type.

DSL — Digital Subscriber Line. One of the latest options for a fast *Internet* connection through existing telephone lines. *Bandwidth* can be very high (1.5 to 9 million Bps). *Upload* speeds usually do not need to be fast as *download* speeds for home applications (most people download much more than they upload), so a less expensive version known as ADSL (asymmetric DSL) is available. This has an upload speed of about 128,000 Bps.

E-mail — Electronic mail. A text-based communications system in which users send and receive documents using the Internet and dedicated e-mail *servers*. Files containing formatted text, images, or sound may be attached to e-mail messages. Each user has a unique e-mail address, which corresponds to a specific mail account with the mail server on a host computer. The address is in the format <<user's account name>>@<<mail server domain name>>.

FAQ — Frequently asked question list. A document that answers the most commonly asked questions about a given topic.

Firewall — A system by which a company or other institution protects itself from unwanted Web traffic. This can prevent outsiders from accessing material within the firewall (eg, to keep out hackers), or it can prevent employees from using the Web for unauthorized purposes (such as playing games).

FTP — File transfer protocol. A way of moving files between computers using the *Internet* (see *http*).

GIF — Graphic interchange format. A way of compressing image files so that they are smaller and better for Internet use. GIF files can save space by reducing the number of colors used to display an image, and hence the number of bits required to describe each pixel, down to a fairly small *palette*. This format is best for cartoons and line drawings with a limited color range, relatively straight edges, and little shading. Photographic images are more commonly stored as *JPEGs*.

Hit — A single request for a file from a Web *server*. This term is used to measure traffic on a *Web site*, but it can be inexact. For example, if your *Web page* has text but no images, a hit may refer to a single visitor viewing the page. If the page has five images on it and some text, when someone visits the sites and sees those elements, six hits will be registered on your *host*. Thus, simply counting hits may overestimate the actual *traffic*. On the other hand, some services (such as America Online) will cache, or copy, your page onto their *server* the first time one of their members requests it. After that, subsequent visitors from that service will get the page from their *server* and not from yours. Therefore, all the subsequent *traffic* from the users of this service will not be registered with your host (until their *server* cache is cleaned out at intervals). In this case, the number of hits may underestimate the actual traffic. A better representation of the number of people who view a *Web site* is the number of unique visitors, a more difficult number to calculate.

Home Page (or Homepage) — (1) The *Web page* displayed by your *browser* when it starts up. (2) The main page of a *Web site*, which is displayed first.

Host — (Noun) A computer that is connected to a network and can be used by individuals connected to the network. A common type of host is a Web *server*. (Verb) To provide space on a *host* computer for a *Web site* or other Internet resource.

HTML — Hypertext markup language. A generic language that is commonly used to write *Web pages*. It specifies the appearance of the page using code elements known as tags. Ideally, a *Web page* should look the same on any computer, regardless of operating system or *browser* software.

HTTP — Hypertext transfer protocol. A way of transferring files over the Internet, commonly used to send Web pages (see *FTP*).

Internet — The collection of approximately 72 million *host* computers (as of mid-2000) that are connected together by a worldwide *network* of cables, telephone lines, satellite links, and other hardware, and that can potentially communicate using a computer "language" known as *TCP/IP*. An analogy would be the worldwide community of English-speaking people, all of whom can potentially communicate given the appropriate physical connection.

internet — A connection between two or more individual *networks* using a common communications protocol. Note the lowercase "i" in the generic version of the word.

Intranet — A network that is very similar to the Internet, but that is limited to a single organization (such as a school or a business), and cannot be accessed from outside that organization.

IP Address — Internet Protocol address. Four numbers, up to three digits each, connected by periods. This is the true address of a computer connected to the *Internet*, and is used by *host* computers to route information to the correct location.

ISDN — Integrated Services Digital Network. A method of providing high-speed *Internet* access over regular phone lines. This is now being supplanted in many areas by *DSL*, which can be significantly faster.

ISP — Internet Service Provider. An entity that supplies access to the Internet through a variety of *network* arrangements. Usually, this is a commercial organization that owns one or more host computers that are connected directly to the Internet. Business and home users rent accounts with the ISP, and are given access to *e-mail*, the *Web*, and a variety of other *Internet* applications. *Web site* hosting may or may not be included in the monthly fee.

Java — A programming language developed by Sun Microsystems. Java programs are designed to run on any computer, and are automatically *downloaded* from *Web sites* to run on the visitor's computer.

JavaScript — A programming language (not to be confused with *Java*). JavaScript was developed by Netscape. It is used in Web site design to add interactive features.

JPEG — Joint Photographic Experts Group. A way of compressing image files to save space. This is commonly used on *Web sites* to reduce download time. JPEG compression is better for photographic images, but *GIF* is preferable for drawings and other images with a relatively small range of colors and sharp, well-defined edges.

LAN — Local area *network*. A *network* that is physically confined to one location, usually a single office or building. See *WAN*.

Link — A part of a *Web page* that acts as a "hot spot." When you click on it, the *browser* then goes to a different *Internet* resource and displays a new *Web page*.

Listserv — One type of *mailing lis*t software, developed by L-soft international, Inc. Frequently used generically to refer to a *mailing list*. Another type of software used for this purpose is Majordomo.

Mailing List — A system that enables people to subscribe to a list based on a topic of common interest, and then to share all *e-mail* sent to the list. By sending *e-mail* to the mailing list address, it will be forwarded to all members of the group.

MIME — Multipurpose Internet mail extension. A standard way of attaching files to *e-mail* (such as images, formatted word processing files, sound files, and so on). If an *e-mail* program is MIME-compliant, it will be able to interpret the attached file regardless of the type of computer that sent the original message. Outside the setting of e-mail, the MIME standards can be used to help *browsers* determine which software is needed to display a variety of file types encountered on the Web.

Modem — MODulator DEModulator. A device that converts digital data into an encoded string of sounds, which are then sent over a telephone connection to another modem, where they are converted back into digital data. This is the most common method of connecting to the *Internet* from home. Most modern analog modems used in *dial-up* accounts are 56K, capable of sending and receiving up to 56,000 *Bps* (rarely achieved in real-world conditions).

Network — The connection of two or more computers (or other devices) in such a way that information can be shared. There are a large number of ways that networks can be constructed, and they can be physically small (two computers in a room sharing a printer), or spread out over thousands of miles (as in dedicated connections between academic, business, or defense computers that bypass the *Internet*). A network consists of a physical connection (such as dedicated cables, wireless transmission, or telephone lines) and a communications *protocol* for the sharing of information. See *LAN, WAN*.

Newsgroup — A "bulletin board"–style arrangement in which topics of common interest are defined and users are allowed to post messages that are read by others in the group. Topics range from the extremely technical (eg, sci.physics.fusion), to the medical (eg, alt.support.arthritis), to the bizarre (eg, alt.jell-o.fetish). The network of these newsgroups is known as USENET.

Online Presence — A representation of a person, business, or other organization on the Internet, typically a *Web site*.

Palette — The range of colors contained in an image. The larger the palette, the more subtle the shading differences that can be represented. A palette can be either a system palette, with a standard set of colors, or an adaptive palette, with colors representing those found in a given image. The adaptive palette allows for more subtle shading of images with a narrow color range without using very large files.

Pathway (Path name) — The location of a file on a computer, usually specified as a hierarchical address within the nested array of folders.

Pixel — Picture element. The smallest unit of an image, represented by a single point on a computer screen or a print. Each point on a computer screen is actually made up of three points in the primary colors. The color of that pixel is determined by the relative contribution of each color. The resolution (or detail level) of an image is typically given in pixels per inch, also known as dots per inch (DPI).

PNG — Short for *portable network graphics*. A nonproprietary alternative to the *GIF* format that allows for image compression and better-quality images. PNG was created to address issues of licensing restrictions associated with the *GIF* format. It has the advantages of supporting *color depth* up to 24 *bits*, and does not lose detail on compression (it is a "lossless" compression scheme, as opposed to *JPEG*, which is "lossy"). PNG has been accepted by the *World Wide Web* consortium on standards, and is becoming more common on the *Internet.*

Portal — A *Web site* that is designed to provide people with frequently requested information in one place, as well as customized links to other sites. Portals commonly include such features as *search engines, directories*, news stories, weather, and sports scores. The purveyors of portals expect that these sites will be the first place that a user goes when logging on to the Internet, making space on their pages a valuable advertising property.

Protocol — A set of standards for communication between computers, analogous to a human language.

Registry — An organization responsible for allocating *domain names* and *IP addresses,* and maintaining the *DNS* database.

Router — A computer that controls traffic across an *internet* by monitoring the addresses to which data are sent on the *networks* and directing it accordingly.

Search Engine — A Web tool that employs a program known as a "*spider*" or "*crawler*" to systematically catalogue a large number of *Web sites* and assemble a database. When a user sends a search request (in the form of one or more keywords), the engine searches the database for matching Web sites, and then displays them in an order determined by the ranking mechanism.

Server — A computer that provides information over a network. A Web server provides pages for the *World Wide Web*, a DNS server provides *IP addresses* in response to *domain names*, while a mail server would receive, store, and distribute *e-mail*.

Spam — Unwanted messages (such as advertisements) that are sent over an *e-mail* system or other communications medium.

Spider — A program that automatically visits sites on the Web to index them for *search engines*.

Surfing — The process of following links from *Web site* to *Web site*.

T-1, T-3 — Dedicated *Internet* connections that are leased, usually to large businesses. They provide stable, high-speed, two-way communication, and may cost thousands of dollars a month to rent. The T-1 line carries 1.5 million *Bps*, and the T-3 carries 44.7 million *Bps*.

TCP/IP — Transmission control protocol/Internet protocol. The method of communication (*protocol*) used by computers connected to the *Internet*.

Telnet — A way of accessing a remote *host* over the Internet, as if one were working on a terminal attached directly to the *host* computer.

Top Level Domain — See *domain name*.

Traffic — Visitors to a *Web site*.

Upload — Transfer of information from a *client* system to a *host* computer.

URL — Uniform resource locator. A standard for describing the location of any Internet resource, including *Web pages*, remote computers (*telnet*), *newsgroups*, or *FTP* sites.

Virtual Address — A *domain name* that does not refer to a single physical computer, but rather to a section of a computer designated to act as an independent addressable entity as seen by the rest of the *Internet* community. If the files of interest are moved to a new location on a different computer, the *DNS* database is simply adjusted to reflect the new *hosting* site, but no change is apparent to those visiting the site.

VRML — Virtual reality markup language. A Web page authoring language that allows for the creation of virtual, three-dimensional worlds, which can be "walked through."

WAN — Wide area network. A network that links together physically distant locations, as might be constructed to ensure reliable communications between military or corporate installations without relying on the *Internet*.

Web Page — A file written in a markup language such as *HTML*, which may contain text as well as links to images, sound, video, animations, and other Web pages. It is displayed for the user on a *browser*.

Web Site — A group of one or more *Web pages*, usually on a single computer, that is organized around a common topic or entity. The pages are held together by internal links.

Web Ring (or Webring) — A series of *Web sites* about a common topic, linked together sequentially, with the last one in the chain then being linked to the first. By using such a ring, a Web user interested in a particular subject can take a "tour" of a number of sites dedicated to that subject.

World Wide Web, WWW, Web — A subset of the Internet in which over a billion pages of text, images, sound, video, and animations are joined together using a vast array of links. *Web pages* are generally written in a standard generic language (see *HTML, XML, VRML, DHTML*) that encodes the appearance of the page so that it is displayed as intended on any type of computer system.

XML — Extensible markup language. A new type of language for creating Web pages. XML enables programmers to define new types of tags, adding functions as needed, as opposed to using a predefined set as in *HTML*. Not all browsers support XML.

Index

D

E

F

G

H

I

J

K

L

M

N

O

P

R

S

T

U

V

W

Y